CW01269360

'Zowie! One of my favourite herbal authors hits a home run again! I didn't know you could do so many things with herbs. Pip Waller stretches the herbal imagination!'

MATTHEW WOOD, herbalist and author of *The Book of Herbal Wisdom*

'Another wonderful, very useful, and incredibly beautiful book from Pip Waller.'

STEPHEN BUHNER, herbalist, earth poet and award-winning author of *The Lost Language of Plants*

'Pip, a successful and experienced herbalist, has put together a wonderful compendium of her own and her colleagues' favourite recipes.'

ELIOT COWAN, founder of the Blue Deer Center, New York, and author of *Plant Spirit Medicine*

'This is an amazing resource full of recipes for a wide variety of daily living and healing products. Great for our health and the environment! I recommend it to anyone who wants to live well and develop a deeper relationship with the products that they use.'

MICHAEL VERTOLLI, founder of the Living School of Herbalism, Canada

'This book of recipes has many gems, which will delight everyone from experienced professional herbalists to herb-loving beginners. A truly creative and inspirational book.'

LUCY HARMER, author of *Shamanic Astrology*

'Having known Pip for approaching thirty years, her on-going commitment to herbal medicine and health care is as fervent now as it was then. Drawing on her own and colleagues' knowledge, *The Domestic Alchemist* offers a practical, encyclopaedic guide on how to make, prepare and use home remedies.'

STEVE KIPPAX, former president of the National Institute of Medical Herbalists

'This essential compendium will delight and excite each and every reader, whether they are a herbalist or have a more general interest in the subject. It is an indispensible guide with easy to follow recipes and lovely illustrations. A must-have text for anyone interested in domestic alchemy.'

DEDJ LEIBBRANDT, fellow of the National Institute of Medical Herbalists

The
DOMESTIC
ALCHEMIST

— 501 —

*Herbal Recipes for
Home, Health & Happiness*

PIP WALLER

Leaping Hare Press

*For Krishna, who is "the potency of medicinal herbs,
the dearest well-wishing friend, the inexhaustible seed."* BG.9.16.

First published in the UK in 2015 by

Leaping Hare Press

210 High Street, Lewes
East Sussex BN7 2NS, UK
www.leapingharepress.co.uk

Text copyright © Pip Waller 2015
Design and layout copyright © Ivy Press Limited 2015

All rights reserved. No part of this book may be reproduced
or transmitted in any form or by any means, electronic, or
mechanical, including photocopying, recording, or by any
information storage-and-retrieval system, without written
permission from the copyright holder.

British Library Cataloguing-in-Publication Data
A catalogue record for this book is available from the British Library

ISBN: 978-1-78240-143-8

This book was conceived, designed and produced by

Leaping Hare Press

Creative Director Peter Bridgewater
Publisher Susan Kelly
Commissioning Editor Monica Perdoni
Art Director Wayne Blades
Senior Editor Jayne Ansell
Designer Andrew Milne

Printed in China

Colour origination by Ivy Press Reprographics

Distributed worldwide (except North America) by
Thames & Hudson Ltd., 181A High Holborn, London WC1V 7QX,
United Kingdom

2 4 6 8 10 9 7 5 3 1

While the publisher and author have made every effort to ensure that the information contained in this book is accurate and presented in good faith, no warranty is provided nor results guaranteed. The publishers and author exclude liability to the fullest extent of the law for any consequence resulting from reliance upon the information contained herein. Readers should always consult a qualified medical practitioner or therapist before undertaking a new diet or health programme.

CONTENTS

Chapter 1
THE POWER OF PLANTS   6

Chapter 2
SOURCING HERBS   10
PICKING HERBS IN THE WILD   11
GROWING HERBS   12

Chapter 3
KITCHEN SET-UP   14
KEY PRESERVATION TECHNIQUES   15
HOW TO USE THIS BOOK SUCCESSFULLY   23

THE RECIPES   24
HOUSEHOLD PRODUCTS   26
ECO-LAUNDRY PRODUCTS   40
KEEPING WELL   52
FIRST-AID PLANT POWER   78
KITCHEN PHARMACY   94
FOOD & DRINK   140
BEAUTY, BALMS & PERSONAL CARE   178
VARIOUS ODDITIES   214

HERB DIRECTORY   222

Contributors   244
Sources & Further Reading   247
Index   248
Acknowledgements   256

Chapter One

The Power of Plants

HERBAL LORE BELONGS TO US ALL, A GREAT AND LASTING LEGACY. Throughout history and across cultures, plants have been used for food, shelter, clothes and medicine. Plants contain the proteins and other nutrients that all animals need to thrive, so we depend on them for our survival. The soil itself is nourished by living plants, and even when they die they decompose to form earth from which new plants can grow. Plants sustain all life; everything we need can be obtained from plants.

Today, however, the central role plants play in human lives has been almost forgotten in the Western world. After several generations of urbanized living, those in modern industrialized countries are far removed from nature, creating a damaging imbalance and further misuse of our greatest resource. Even most of us living in rural areas no longer regularly cultivate, gather and use the helpful plants that grow all around us.

ALCHEMISTS OF THE NATURAL WORLD

Herbs are the wondrous 'alchemists' of the natural world. They take carbon dioxide from the atmosphere for their energy production, and give back the oxygen that we need to breathe; they take nitrogen from the air and use it to make amino acids, the building blocks of proteins. Plants build all kinds of chemicals, and they do so in constant relationship to the circumstances in which they find themselves, and in communication with each other. They make medicines – for themselves, for other plants, for the soil and environment around them, and for us.

NATURAL MEDICINE

Herbal medicine has been the mainstay and root of medicine from earliest times. In some ancient tombs, archaeologists have discovered the remains of plants still known to herbalists for their power to treat conditions such as arthritis, which modern science has detected in the bodies they accompany. Every culture and every land has a rich history of herbal medicine. Even up to the present day, many drugs used in modern medicine come from plant-based sources.

My own interest in herbal medicine grew in the 1980s when both my parents suffered from health problems. At the time, using anything other than conventional medicine was almost unheard of, and any mention of alternative medicine was met with a doubtful 'Does it actually work?' My parents were concerned about the implications of medicines our regular doctor was suggesting, though, and decided to approach a herbalist for advice. They began taking herbal remedies routinely and the results were incredible – my father was even able to avoid surgery. I was impressed, and so drawn to the subject that I went on to study herbal medicine at the School of Phytotherapy in Kent, and joined The National Institute of Medical Herbalists.

A NEW PERSPECTIVE

I began to learn about herbalism's rich heritage, and its success in curing all kinds of problems. During the great cholera epidemic of the nineteenth century, for example, many herbalists in industrial towns became famous for rarely losing a patient; and following the disastrous explosion at Chernobyl, the Soviet nuclear plant, in 1986, it was found that growing comfrey lowered levels of radiation poisoning in the surrounding soil. This knowledge fascinated me, and I continue to be enlightened.

The more I experience and learn about the power of plants, the more baffled I am that herbalism is sometimes still regarded as being paradoxically 'ineffective' on the one hand and 'dangerous' on the other. I wanted to write a book that would help dispel these myths and encourage readers to start their own lifelong journey of discovery into herbalism.

HARMONY & HAPPINESS

'Wood warms you three times – first when you gather it, second when you chop it, and third when you burn it.'
Similarly, making your own plant-based recipes for home and health provides three sources of happiness and relaxation:

First, being outside in nature gathering plants or tending pot herbs on your windowsill, drying and preparing those you have grown, even enjoying measuring out dried herbs and oils bought in for potion making; all connect us to nature which brings harmony and balance into our lives. In fact, feeling your inherent connection to the natural world will bring inestimable happiness.

Second, pottering around in your kitchen laboratory is great fun. You will embark on an empowering journey of exploration as you discover herbs and concoct unique recipes for your home, health and happiness.

Third, when you use the magical elixir you have made, or share it with a friend, you will feel a tremendous sense of satisfaction.

In short, plants contribute to our happiness and well-being in so many different ways; their inherent usefulness isn't the only joy they bring.

CONNECTING WITH THE NATURAL WORLD

This is a book for anyone with an interest in using plants in the home – for herbalists and kitchen herbalists, for conservationists, for anyone with even a passing interest in herbs. It's a book for those looking to live a more natural life, to welcome the spirit and usefulness of the plant world into their lives and to connect with the natural world – whether you live in a semi-rural location (as I do) or a city apartment.

The 501 recipes in this book have been gathered by myself over many years as a herbalist, and include contributions from experts across the United States, Canada, the UK and Europe. They range from teas to meads, from toothpastes to face masks, from laundry detergent to air freshener. Some are very simple, requiring almost no equipment; others are complex, such as cream blending, soap making or distilling aromatic waters. My hope is that as your confidence grows, you will begin to experiment and create your own variations. The next few pages of this book are dedicated to showing you all that you need to start your plant-based preparations at home. They include equipment that you will require, information on sourcing and storing herbs and some key techniques for preserving herbs.

Plants are truly life-enhancing, and herbalism, and the love and appreciation of nature that it fosters, is for everyone. I hope this book helps to lead you on a rich journey of discovery.

Chapter Two
Sourcing Herbs

SOURCING HERBS NEEDS A LITTLE THOUGHT. Whether you choose to pick herbs in the wild, grow your own or buy them in, you will need a certain amount of background knowledge. The following pages are dedicated to providing a few guidelines, and the Herb Directory on pages 222–243 can also be used as a starting point to help identify and source plants.

Even if you begin by buying in all your ingredients, I hope that as your confidence grows you will be inspired to take a step further and discover living plants in nature. Native wisdom from all over the world states that local herbs are many times more effective than those grown at a distance. It is known that plants adapt their chemistry to their environment.

The feeling of connection that a human can have with the plant world is irreplaceable in its health-giving and balancing propensity. When you get to know living plants, you will begin to see friends everywhere you go.

PICKING HERBS IN THE WILD

Foraging, or wildcrafting, is increasingly popular, and you need not live in the woods to do it. It's amazing how many useful herbs grow in the nooks and crannies of a city. When gathering from the wild, there are a few important considerations.

Firstly, treat the environment with respect and don't over-forage. A good guideline is to always take a little under half of what is there – and if the plant is endangered, don't take any at all. If you are gathering the root of a plant, or a whole plant (as opposed to just some flowers, leaves, stems or bark), then plant some seeds or a new plant. With some plants, you can divide the roots and replant half again.

Secondly, check for contamination. In farming areas, avoid land that has been crop sprayed, especially very recently. In cities, find out the previous use of waste land, making sure it wasn't used for toxic chemical production, dumping or such like. It's also important to take care that you are not trespassing on private land, and to check out local laws about gathering plants.

Plant identification is an invaluable skill, and there are excellent books with clear photographs to help the lone learner. If you take this route, you must be extremely careful not to use the wrong plant: if you're not sure, leave it be. While few plants are seriously poisonous, some can harm and even kill you if taken by mistake. There are useful resources online about foraging; I have included some at the back of this book.

Before I pick, I follow the native tradition of asking the plant's permission in my heart (respecting a 'no' if I feel I hear one), and offering gratitude and something in return. In America, the traditional offering is tobacco; in Europe, it is oats or barley. Even if this seems strange to you, I encourage you to try it. You may be surprised at the warmth it will bring you. The earth is a living treasury, and the more you recognize its offerings, the richer your life will be.

GROWING HERBS

Plants, generally, are easy to please – they like enough (but not too much) light, water and food, and the right kind of earth. They also respond to love: talking to your plants and caring for them actually makes them grow more abundantly. This attitude can be even more important than the quality of the earth in which they are grown, as shown by the famous eco-community of Findhorn, near Forres in Scotland, who have grown impossibly enormous vegetables on soil that was little more than earth-covered rock.

You can grow some herbs anywhere. They are ideal for urban settings and don't require a lot of space; many thrive in a windowbox or containers as well as planted in the ground. A lot of herbs – 'herbs' being the general word for describing plants used in medicine, or to give flavour and texture in cooking – are very easy to grow.

Many plants love a bit of attention. The more you pick the flowers of the marigold, for example, the more it will flower. And most plants prefer a sheltered spot and the company of other plants. Check for any individual requirements of the herbs you grow, and grow them simply, using organic or bio methods, for maximum benefit.

Start growing whatever takes your fancy, and whatever you can easily find. You can sow seeds – try marigold (*Calendula officinalis*), nasturtium and Californian poppy as a few very easy starters. Or buy small plants to start you off, such as oregano or marjoram, or thyme. I grow a stevia plant (a great natural sweetener) on my bathroom windowsill where it keeps coming year after year; I keep cutting the stems to use in recipes, and more grow back. Every couple of years I re-pot it carefully to give it some fresh earth. I tried to grow this plant in the kitchen for a while, but the steaminess in the bathroom seems to suit her more.

Make inquiries locally to see what grows well in your area, and just have a go. Make friends with local gardeners – they will give you tips, and probably some plants to start you off. Try planting things inside or out: if they are happy, continue as you are; if not, try something else! You are likely to be pleasantly occupied and very satisfied with your home-grown results.

PICKING HERBS

Harvest plants on a fine day, picking leaves and flowers around mid-morning when the dew has dried. Remember to take a small pocketknife. Keep an eye on the plants you want so that you can pick them at their peak. Choose the healthiest plants/parts of plants. If you plan to use them fresh in a recipe, try to pick and use immediately.

DRYING & STORING HERBS

Wash plants if necessary, then remove and compost unhealthy or unnecessary parts. Gather the aerial parts (those above ground) into a bundle and tie up at the bottom of the stems, or put them into a paper bag. Hang the bundle or bag in a warm, well-ventilated place, indoors or out. Herbs take up to several days to dry depending on conditions.

All parts of plants can be spread out in single layers on trays to dry in a warm, well-ventilated place. Use mesh trays or trays lined with fresh tea towels or paper. Turn the plant matter daily to encourage even drying. Roots can be left whole or roughly chopped (it's easier to cut them fresh). Flowers and leaves are easier to remove from stems when dry. You can also dry plant material in a dehumidifier.

Aim to dry the plant material enough to stop it going mouldy, without taking all the life away. Store your dried plants in paper bags sealed from the air, or in airtight jars, and keep away from direct sunlight. If dried well, herbs will keep with full properties for at least a year. After this, they will not be as beneficial.

Buying In

What cannot be grown or foraged can be bought in, choosing organically grown ingredients as much as possible. Be responsible when buying wildcrafted herbs, and make sure they were properly picked with sustainability in mind. Reputable suppliers of herbs can be found easily online, and you may be lucky and have a good herbal shop near enough to visit. Find a local herbal practitioner and ask his or her advice about local suppliers. This also puts you in touch with a qualified professional to consult when you need to.

When you are buying herbs in a relatively raw state – for example, dried to use in a recipe – you will easily be able to tell the quality by looking, smelling and tasting a little.

Some of the recipes in this book include ingredients you will need to buy in. All of these are readily available.

Chapter Three

Kitchen Set-up

VERY LITTLE SPECIAL EQUIPMENT IS NEEDED to start creating useful, plant-based preparations at home, but you will want to prepare your working area and acquire a few necessary items before you start to gather your herbs. The basic kit on pages 16–17 lists essential pieces of equipment and explains how these are used. The recipes in this book assume you have this basic kit, noting only additional 'speciality' items not on this list.

Before you move on to the recipe section, you will need some knowledge of the key techniques herbalists use to extract and preserve a herb's wonderful properties. The following pages are dedicated to this, and you will be referred back to this section frequently during the course of the book.

KEY PRESERVATION TECHNIQUES

A domestic alchemist can extract and preserve the properties he or she needs from plants in various ways. The materials you choose will affect the quality of the final product. Try to choose organically grown ingredients wherever possible, and use raw (unpasteurized) honey and apple cider vinegar for anything taken inside the body. Water used for making any preparation should be of good quality; unless you have access to pure spring water, filtered is best, being both cleaner than average tap water and more environmentally friendly than bottled water.

HERBAL INFUSIONS

Leaves and flowers as well as ground roots and barks can be made into infusions (also called teas or tisanes). These can be prepared with fresh or dried herbs.

Hot Infusions

Unless instructed otherwise, teas in this book are to be made as follows:

Place 1 tsp dried herb material or 2 tsp fresh in a teapot or pan with a lid. Cover with a mug of boiling water and leave with a lid on to infuse or brew for 10 minutes. Strain before use.

If a stronger tea is required, the traditional dose is 25g/1oz dried herb or double the quantity of fresh steeped in 550ml/2⅓ cups water. Some recipes call for these stronger herbal infusions.

Cold Infusions

Cold infusions are made by steeping herbs in cold water for 2–3 hours. They are usually made with fresh flowers and leaves.

Decoctions

Parts of the plant that are tougher (such as roots and barks) need to be boiled in water. This is known as a 'decoction', though it can also be called a tea. Decoctions can be made with similar amounts as the teas above, but a little extra water is added to allow for evaporation while simmering. In making decoctions, the plant matter is put into a saucepan with water, covered with a lid, heated and then simmered for 10–15 minutes.

After the infusion or decoction is made, usually (but not always) the liquid is strained off and the solid plant matter discarded (for composting). If the liquid is being used in an eye bath or a cream, it should be strained through a sieve lined with muslin or thin cotton cloth (p.16) to ensure absolutely no bits remain.

Infusions and decoctions can be drunk hot or cold, applied externally as lotions or washes and used in the making of other preparations, such as creams. They keep for 3 days in the fridge. If you bottle them hot into sterilized bottles (p.17), you can keep the unopened bottles for up to a month.

Aromatic Waters

It is exciting to turn a tea or decoction from an aromatic herb into a 'water', which involves distillation. A simple method using an adapted pressure cooker is described with the recipes. Aromatic waters can keep for anywhere between 3 months and 2 years.

BASIC KIT

RACK, STRING, PAPER BAGS, SELECTION OF GLASS JARS AND STORAGE CONTAINERS, LABELS
Freshly picked herbs can be tied together and hung from a rack to dry. When dried, store in paper bags or glass jars with tightly fitting lids, away from direct sunlight.

Jars are also used to store tinctures, vinegars and infused oils; you may want large ones for this purpose – old sweet jars work well. Small jars are useful for storing creams; bottles for liquid preparations. You may also need old shampoo bottles and so forth, plus spray bottles and dropper bottles. Almost everything you make will need a label.

Whatever you use to store your preparations needs to be very clean. It is absolutely essential to sterilize bottles or jars used for storing syrups, glycerine, tinctures, jellies, creams and ointments (see box, opposite).

COFFEE GRINDER
For grinding dried herbs and roots. Ground herbs are used in infusions, oil blends, chocolates, snuff, scouring powder, medicines and foods.

TEAPOT OR COVERED PAN (OR A TEA INFUSER IF FOR ONE PERSON)
For brewing infusions (herbal teas).

FUNNELS
For pouring and straining. You need both large and small, to fit the necks of storage bottles.

MUSLINS OR THIN COTTON CLOTH
For straining potions. Use squares of muslin, large cotton handkerchiefs or tea towels.

SIEVES AND STRAINERS
Metal sieves, from tea-strainer size upwards, are useful for straining. (A small wine press, of the kind normally used for home brewing, is good for pressing out tinctures, infused oils, etc.)

KITCHEN SET-UP

COOKING IMPLEMENTS
For brewing up mixtures, use pots, pans, heat-resistant stainless steel or silicone spatulas and spoons, and a potato masher.

DOUBLE BOILER/BAIN-MARIE
For heating potions gently, use a stainless steel double boiler or a 'bain-marie' – a baking dish or saucepan half-filled with water on the stove top, with heat-resistant bowls containing your potions inside it.

MEASURING EQUIPMENT
A couple of accurate measuring jugs, cups and spoons for measuring ingredients. For medicinal tincture mixtures, use a 100ml measuring cylinder.

DIGITAL SCALES
Some recipes require accurately weighed ingredients.

Sterilizing

It is very important to sterilize equipment properly before preserving any plant material, as failure to do so will not only lessen the shelf-life of your product but could also potentially cause food poisioning.

Sterilize items immediately before use. Cool jars/bottles first for cold preparations, but always pour hot preparations (jellies, hot oils, syrups etc.) into hot jars or bottles. You can sterilize items in a number of ways:

1 Remove any plastic lids and cook clean glass bottles and jars in the oven (140°C/275°F/Gas Mark 1) for 20–30 minutes.

2 Boil in water for 10 minutes (boil lids separately). Keep bottles and lids covered by water until just before use.

3 Use a microwave or dishwasher – check the manufacturer's instructions before proceeding.

HERBAL TINCTURES

Plants' qualities can be extracted and preserved using alcohol. Tinctures, as they are known, were traditionally made by boiling herbs in wine, but are now produced by steeping the herb in a solution of alcohol and water. Herbalists use variable concentrations of alcohol for different plants, from solutions of 15–25 per cent up to 90 per cent alcohol for resins. (These are substances exuded from certain trees, many of which have strong antiseptic and healing properties, such as myrrh.)

Producing tinctures at home usually means using shop-bought alcoholic spirits. Always aim to use organic spirits. The best one is vodka because it has little taste, though any strong spirit will do. Vodka is usually about 40 per cent alcohol.

If you are making a tincture with fresh plant material (called a 'specific tincture'), the water in the plant will even things out nicely down to a tincture of around 25–30 per cent proof. If you are using dried herbs, though, you may want to add 85ml/⅓ cup water to dilute each 200ml/just over ¾ cup alcohol. Alternatively, dilute with an infusion or decoction of the herb, which gives you a combination of tea and tincture in one remedy.

Make tinctures by covering plant material with between two and five times the amount of alcohol solution in a large jar with a well-fitting lid. It is best to use weights for the amount of herb used. A general guide could be 200g/7oz dried herb (300g/10½oz fresh) to each 1 litre/1 quart alcohol solution.

Leave to stand in a cool, dark place for at least 3 weeks, turning upside down or shaking the jar once a day. (Many traditions encourage talking or singing to the plants as you do this.) After 3–8 weeks, strain the liquid through a sieve or funnel lined with thin cloth. Pull the edges of the cloth up and around the macerated herbs, then twist, wring and press it to extract all of the liquid. Store in a clean bottle.

Fluid extracts are tinctures made with equal amounts of plant material to alcohol. They can be made by double infusing (p.20).

Tinctures are used in creams, lotions and liniments, or taken internally. Even a small dose of tincture is effective.

Some herbalists work entirely with drop doses, and some herbs are only taken in drop doses (e.g. 5–20 drops, 1–3 times daily); always use drop doses for children. Many herbalists use a standard adult dose of 5ml/1 tsp mixed in 30ml/2 tbsp hot or cold water, taken once a day for a tonic or preventative or 3 times a day for chronic ailments. For acute conditions, 5–10ml/1–2 tsp can be taken 3–6 times daily.

Tinctures are often mixed together in blends; there are many recipes for blends in this book. You can either buy in the tinctures to make them or produce your own, using the guidelines above. For these blends, herbalists tend to use only millilitres (ml) as measurements, as this is the easiest and best way. You can make them with teaspoon measures (1 tsp = 5ml, 1 tbsp = 15ml), but it is quite fiddly. If you are regularly making these mixtures, I suggest you buy a 100ml plastic measuring cylinder (they cost about £1.50).

Not everyone can tolerate, or wishes to take, alcohol, in which case tinctures can be made with the same quantities of glycerine.

Many leading herbalists tailor-make tinctures each time, rather than using standard amounts; as the American herbalist Matthew Wood, author of *The Book of Herbal Wisdom* (1997), explains: 'I look for the distinctive taste of every plant in the extract. Therefore, I make the tincture to the "right taste" … I prefer to think of tinctures and other preparations by analogy to wine, not to pharmaceutical drugs.'

Tinctures can also be made into delicious alcoholic beverages that are pleasant to drink and have health-giving properties in small doses. These can be made with wine, mead (my personal favourite) or with any spirit: gin (sloe gin is the famous one), brandy, vodka, rum, whisky, if you like it, or the local home-distilled schnapps. Usually, a little honey or sugar is added while the tincture is steeping, otherwise the method is the same.

Kept in a cool place away from the sun, a well-made tincture will keep for at least 2 years, some many more.

HERBAL VINEGARS

Vinegars are a useful medium for extracting and preserving herbs; they are used in foods, taken as supplements or medicines and used in many home cleaning products and hair and skin tonics.

Vinegar, especially raw (unpasteurized) organic apple cider vinegar, is good for you inside and out. Taken internally, it can encourage a healthy pH balance, reduce inflammation, boost immunity and regularize metabolism. Taken with food, it enables you to absorb minerals better. Externally, it can bring bruises to the surface, cool and reduce swellings, and benefit the hair and skin.

Herbal vinegars are made like tinctures. Steep the herb in 2–3 times the amount of vinegar. Leave for 2–4 weeks in a cool, dark place, then strain through cloth. As medicines, the dose is the same as for tinctures (see opposite). Vinegars can keep for at least 2 years.

COMPRESS & POULTICE

Vinegars, tinctures and teas can be used to make a compress. Soak a cloth in the herb liquid, lay it, heated or cold, against the skin and secure with a suitable bandage. It will help to soothe aches and pains, sore throats, headaches and skin conditions.

Fresh plant material can be used to make poultices – mashed or crushed herbs applied to the body alone. Poultices can stay in place for 2–3 days, though many choose to replace them daily.

OXYMELS

An oxymel is a tasty remedy that combines the healing properties of a herbal vinegar with honey – itself a miraculous substance, known to be antibiotic and encouraging to the immune system. Oxymels are made by gently warming a herbal vinegar with an equal amount of honey until the honey is dissolved. In sterile bottles (p.17), oxymels keep for 2 years.

INFUSED OILS

Infused oils, made in the same way as tinctures and vinegars, can be used alone or in ointments, creams, liniments and lotions.

To make, combine 1 part herb with 2–3 parts vegetable oil, then leave for 4–8 weeks to infuse. Note that infused oils are mostly made in the shade, as vegetable oils go off, but some need sunlight to work properly. The recipes in this book will say if sun is required. Once infused, strain and press through cloth, as described for tinctures (p.18).

You can make an infused oil more quickly by gently heating the herb in the oil, usually in a double boiler or 'bain-marie' (p.17), for 2–4 hours.

Many vegetable oils can be used to make a herbal infused oil. The most commonly used include olive, almond, sunflower, coconut, safflower, rapeseed, grapeseed, sesame and jojoba. The base oils all have medicinal properties of their own, and I recommend researching which oil will best offer what you require. Always use the best organically grown, cold-pressed oil that you can afford. Olive oil infusions can keep for up to a year before they start to smell off, and coconut infusions can keep for 2 years, but most others will go off in a few months.

Sometimes a 'double infusion' is made to obtain a higher-strength product. In such cases, the infused oil is made and then used to infuse a fresh quantity of plant material. (This can also be done with tinctures, vinegars and all water-based preparations.)

An infused oil can be made into a salve, balm or ointment by addition of an emulsifier such as beeswax. The more wax you use, the harder the ointment becomes. For a soft salve, 8–10 per cent wax to oil is used.

LINIMENTS

Liniments are warming, stimulating rubs for aches and pains. They rub in very easily and are lighter than an oil, so are useful for covering large areas. Liniments are made by mixing an infused oil and a tincture or vinegar. The two will naturally separate in the bottle, so they need to be shaken before each use. How long a liniment keeps for will depend upon the base oil (e.g. olive oil, almond oil) you're using.

CREAMS

Creams can be quite difficult to make successfully. They mix oil and water components, which require an emulsifier. The purist natural cream maker will use beeswax and a serious amount of whisking instead of a manufactured emulsifier.

To make creams the old-fashioned way, heat the oil and water components separately to a similar temperature using a double boiler or bain-marie (p.17); in a double boiler you can heat the water part in the bottom and the oil in the top. Then pour the water part very slowly into the oil part, whisking furiously. Once the oil and water are mixed, the cream is usually quickly cooled by placing the mixing bowl into a cold bath (a pan of cold water). Usually, you continue to whisk while cooling, and until the cream is formed, then put into sterilized jars.

Using a bought-in emulsifying wax makes cream making a simpler process. This is a substance used in cosmetic manufacturing; you can buy it made from pure vegetable sources, but as it is a 'man-made' ingredient purists tend to spurn it.

How long creams keep for varies greatly. Those made with long-lasting coconut oil, for example, could keep for a year; with some other oils, creams may only last for 1–2 months, unless a preservative is added.

SOAPS

Soap basically consists of vegetable oils that have been saponified (turned into soap) with a strong alkaloid, known as lye. Soap making is easy to pull off successfully; however, it involves a lot of steps and some substances that need handling and measuring very carefully. For this reason, ingredients for soaps are weighed, and you'll need digital scales to make them.

Solid soap is made via a 'cold process' using sodium hydroxide, which involves a lot of stirring and no heat. Liquid soap uses potassium hydroxide in a 'hot process', which involves a lot of stirring and the use of a slow cooker to provide heat. Herbs and essential oils are then added after the oils and lye have been mixed. Soaps keep for years, though they will lose their smell over time as the essential oils evaporate.

SYRUPS, HONEYS & SWEETS

Sugar and honey can be used in various ways to preserve plants. Both can be used to make syrups that are soothing and nourishing, particularly for the throat and chest, and are good for preserving vitamin C.

A simple syrup is made by boiling a 65 per cent sugar and water solution (i.e. one that contains twice the quantity of sugar to liquid) for 3–5 minutes, or by first making a strong infusion or decoction and then boiling this with the sugar.

When making a syrup with raw honey, do not boil, as this destroys its healthful enzymes. Just add an equal amount of honey to a strong herbal decoction or infusion and then heat the mixture gently to dissolve. Infused honeys can also be made simply by mixing the honey and the herbs and leaving to infuse for a few weeks.

Store the syrup in sterilized bottles (p.17), first putting the lids on loosely, then tightening when cold. 65 per cent sugar syrups keep very well. You can also make a 40–50 per cent syrup that will keep fairly well unopened if it is thoroughly sterilized. Syrups tend to go off quickly once opened, so store your syrup in several smaller bottles rather than one large bottle to help improve its shelf-life.

Syrups can also be sterilized again once bottled, to preserve them further. Set the lids on loosely, then place the bottles on layers of paper in a pan (the water should reach three-quarters of the way up the bottles' sides). Simmer the water for 10 minutes, then immediately remove and tighten up the lids.

Sweets are made from a 65 per cent syrup that has been boiled for a long time. Sometimes tinctures and essential oils may be added in at the end. Some recipes use half sugar, half golden syrup.

Boil the syrup for 20–30 minutes to evaporate the water, leaving more and more sugar in the mix. This then goes through several stages. The 'hard-ball' stage, which is the minimum needed for sweets, occurs after this 20–30 minutes, so start testing after 15 minutes. Drop a little of the mix into cold water and watch.

At 'hard-ball' stage, the mixture makes a ball shape; it keep its shape but feels sticky to the touch. The next stage, known as the 'soft-crack' stage, can occur minutes later. The mixture now solidifies into threads that are flexible to the touch and will bend a little before breaking. The third stage, known as the 'hard-crack' stage, occurs minutes after this. At this point the threads break immediately. As the three stages occur in very quick succession, I recommend testing your mixture every few minutes after you reach the 'hard-ball' stage.

Anywhere between 'hard-ball' and 'hard-crack' stage works for herbal sweets; after that you are in burning territory! As the 'hard-ball' stage is sufficient, pour your mix on to a lightly oiled baking tray when you reach this point, scoring both ways to make small tablet shapes as it cools. Alternatively, pour into small moulds and leave to set. If adding essential oils, do this just before pouring out. If adding honey to the mixture, I like to boil it a bit longer until 'hard-crack' stage is reached. Then add the honey just before pouring it out. When the contents are cold, they can be turned out and broken into pieces as necessary.

Keep the sweets in a sealed container in a cool place with some icing sugar, cornflour or ground slippery elm to stop them sticking together. Stored this way, they will last well for 3–4 weeks and up to 6 weeks.

Essential Oils

Essential oils are a valuable addition to many recipes. These are generally bought in, as they are extracted by a complex distillation process; they contain potent properties from the plant, and are used in small quantities. They mix easily in fixed oils, but tend to float on top if mixed in a water preparation, unless emulsified in some way. Mixing the oils with a little vegetable glycerine first can help. Essential oils are volatile and are lost by heating, so are added at the end of any recipes using heat. Some will strip paint or eat into rubber, so if you are experimenting with recipes, bear this in mind and be cautious.

LABELLING & STORING

When you have finished making a product, be sure to label it with what it is and the date made; otherwise you will end up with a shelf full of lovely potions and lotions that you have no idea what to do with!

Unless the recipe says otherwise, store all products in a cool, dark place in an appropriate vessel – a sterilized bottle or jar with a tight-fitting lid, or an airtight container. This will ensure each product keeps at its best for as long as possible. Each recipe includes a recommended shelf-life; this should be used as a guide, with common sense always prevailing. If a product starts smelling odd, discard it.

HOW TO USE THIS BOOK SUCCESSFULLY

There is a wide range of recipes in this book – from tincture blends and infusions to soaps and creams. To make them successfully, there is some important information you need to keep in mind.

INGREDIENTS

- Some recipes are made from fresh herbs, others are bought-in, and some use a mixture. Unless fresh or dried herbs are specified, it should be assumed that you can use *either* fresh or dried herbs for each recipe. If the amounts differ depending on whether you use fresh or dried, this will be stated.

- Many ingredients lists contain pre-made preparations – tinctures, infusions and so on. Where a specific recipe for these appears in the book, you will be referred to it; otherwise, you will be referred back to the key preservations section (pp.15–22) for the standard technique.

EQUIPMENT & METHOD

- Before you start making anything, gather together the basic equipment (pp.16–17). All the recipes assume you have this equipment to hand; only if you need something less common will it be specified.

- Some recipes are very simple and others quite complex. In the interests of space, the various methods are described in full once only, and you will be referred back to this as required. Always carefully read the recipe, and if necessary, the general information found elsewhere in the book, before beginning.

MEASUREMENTS

- Herbalism isn't an exact science. Many herbalists do not work with rote amounts, tending to measure by eye to produce the desired result. With this is mind, most recipes – such as food, cleaners and so on – use rough approximations.

- Some recipes, however, require that ingredients be very carefully weighed – this includes many medicines, all soaps (as you're using caustic substances) and some creams (which can be tricky to make). In such recipes, cup conversions or tablespoon measurements do not provide the necessary accuracy, so they have not been provided and their use is not advised.

- Tablespoon and teaspoon measurements provided in this book are based on the following:
  1 tbsp = 15ml
  1 tsp = 5ml
  ½ tsp = 2.5ml
  I advise using these standard-sized spoons for all recipes that require tablespoon or teaspoon amounts, and for doses.

- Adult doses are provided as standard for all remedies; children take the smaller end of the dose range, or ¼–½ the adult dose, unless otherwise specified. See page 94 for more details on doses, and see the box on page 24, 'Taking Herbal Remedies'.

Taking Herbal Remedies

Herbal remedies can work remarkably well, and sometimes they work fast. Often they are not a quick fix, however, needing instead to be taken over weeks and months to achieve the desired effect. Recipes for medicines depend on empirical, traditional knowledge, some of which (but not all) is backed up by modern scientific research.

Responsibility for self-prescribing any of the remedies in this book falls solely with the reader.

If you are pregnant or breast-feeding, have any serious or long-lasting health condition, or if you are already taking medication, it is especially important to first seek the advice of a healthcare professional.

The Recipes

HOUSEHOLD PRODUCTS

The cleaners in this section are wonderful and effective environmentally friendly alternatives to strong-smelling chemicals. The essential oils leave a fresh clean smell and mildly disinfect the area. Herbs also make perfect room sprays and wonderful potpourri.

Chamomile & Marjoram Surface Cleaner

The addition of chamomile and marjoram gives this gentle but effective eco-cleaner a beautiful, sweet scent.

INGREDIENTS
- 500ml/2 cups distilled white vinegar
- 2 tsp marjoram flowers and leaves
- 1–2 tsp chamomile flower heads
- 20 drops lavender essential oil

MAKES & KEEPS
Makes 500ml/2 cups.
Keeps up to 2 years.

METHOD
Make an infused vinegar with the herbs (p.19). Add the essential oil and decant into a spray bottle (for easy cleaning).

For everyday use, add an equal amount of water to the mixture. Spray on, leave for a few minutes and wipe off.

For really tough jobs, use the cleaner undiluted – gently heating for a few minutes makes it extra strong. Spray dirty surfaces with hot vinegar cleaner and leave for 15 minutes before scrubbing and rinsing.

All-purpose Cleaning Spray

Courtesy of Michael Vertolli

INGREDIENTS
- 200ml/¾ cup + 5 tsp water, boiled or distilled
- 50ml/3 tbsp + 1 tsp distilled white vinegar
- 1 drop Liquid Castile Soap (p.199)

Essential oils:
- 5 drops lavender
- 3 drops pine
- 3 drops spruce or fir
- 1 drop geranium

MAKES & KEEPS
Makes 250ml/1 cup.
Keeps indefinitely.

METHOD
Combine the ingredients in a spray bottle and shake to mix.

Shake well before use. Spray the surface, then wipe clean.

Lemon-fresh Cleaner

INGREDIENTS
- 500ml/2 cups distilled white vinegar
- 1 lemon, sliced

Essential oils:
- 10 drops lemon
- 10 drops orange

MAKES & KEEPS
Makes 500ml/2 cups.
Keeps 1 year or more.

METHOD
Make an infused vinegar with the lemon (p.19), then add the essential oils.

Use as for Chamomile & Marjoram Surface Cleaner (opposite).

Bug-busting Surface Cleaner

INGREDIENTS
- 500ml/2 cups distilled white vinegar
- 1–2 tsp thyme leaves
- 2 tsp marigold petals
- 20 drops thyme essential oil

MAKES & KEEPS
Makes 500ml/2 cups.
Keeps up to 2 years.

METHOD
Make an infused vinegar with the thyme and marigold (p.19), then add the essential oil.

Use as for Chamomile & Marjoram Surface Cleaner (opposite).

Anti-bacterial Multi-surface Cleaner

Courtesy of Teri Evans

INGREDIENTS
- 1 tsp borax (see box, p.43)
- 1 tsp bicarbonate of soda
- 2 tsp lemon juice
- 400ml/1⅔ cups hot water

Essential oils:
- 10 drops tea tree
- 5 drops eucalyptus
- 5 drops lavender

MAKES & KEEPS
Makes approx. 400ml/1⅔ cups.
Keeps up to 2 months.

METHOD
Put all the ingredients in an empty spray cleaner bottle. Shake well to mix, repeating vigorously before each use.

Rinse surfaces after spraying to remove traces of borax and oils.

Zesty Washing-up Liquid

INGREDIENTS
- 4 tsp washing soda
- 375ml/1½ cups boiling water
- 5 tbsp Liquid Castile Soap (p.199) or ¾ of a 250g/9oz bar grated solid castile soap

Essential oils:
- 10 drops lemon or orange
- 10 drops grapefruit
- 10 drops tea tree

MAKES & KEEPS
Makes approx. 425ml/1¾ cups.
Keeps at least 6 months.

METHOD
If using grated soap, stir into the water until dissolved, then slowly stir in the soda. If not, dissolve the washing soda in the water, then add the liquid soap, continuing to stir until dissolved. Leave to cool. When cool, stir in the essential oils and bottle.

Shake well before use.

— *Tip* —

IF YOU USE GRATED SOLID SOAP, YOUR HOMEMADE WASHING-UP LIQUID MAY THICKEN IN THE COLD. USING LESS WASHING SODA WILL GIVE A THINNER LIQUID IF YOU LIVE IN COLDER CLIMES. ALWAYS RINSE WELL AFTER WASHING, AS FOR ANY WASHING-UP LIQUID.

Eco-powered Oven Cleaner with Basil

This is as effective as commercial brands, without the chemicals.

INGREDIENTS
- 120ml/½ cup Liquid Castile Soap (p.199)
- 250g/1¼ cups bicabonate of soda
- 4 tbsp rosemary vinegar (p.19)
- 4 drops basil essential oil (optional)

MAKES & KEEPS
Makes enough for one really thorough clean. Mix the cleaner up freshly each time you need it.

METHOD
Mix all the ingredients thoroughly in a bowl. Remove the oven shelves and clean separately.

Using a paintbrush, spread your mixture over the entire surface of the oven. Leave it for 6–8 hours or overnight. During this time the mixture will foam up slightly and lift the grime from the oven surface.

Using a bowl full of clean water and a damp foam scrubber, wipe out the oven. Change the water as needed. If the oven is really greasy and hasn't been cleaned for a while, repeat the process once more.

Rosemary & Pine Toilet Cleaner

INGREDIENTS
- 1 small handful of rosemary leaves
- 1 large handful of pine needles, removed from the stems
- 500ml/2 cups white or Apple Cider Vinegar (p.165)
- 50 drops/½ tsp rosemary essential oil (optional)
- 50 drops/½ tsp pine essential oil (optional)

MAKES & KEEPS
Makes about 500ml/2 cups.
Keeps at least 1 year.

METHOD
Make an infused vinegar with the fresh rosemary and pine needles (p.19). If desired, add the essential oils for a stronger odour.

Pour a bucket of water down the toilet to force water out of the bowl. This will enable you to reach the sides more easily. Then pour the undiluted cleaner into the bowl and leave for 10–20 minutes. Scrub well with a toilet brush.

Thyme & Marigold Disinfectant

INGREDIENTS
- 500ml/2 cups distilled white vinegar or Apple Cider Vinegar (p.165)
- 100 drops/1 tsp thyme essential oil
- 15g/½oz dried thyme (or 1 handful of freshly picked if possible, the leaves removed from the stems)
- 15g/½oz dried marigold flowers (or 1 handful of fresh)

MAKES & KEEPS
Makes around 450ml/just under 2 cups.
Keeps at least 2 years.

METHOD
Make an infused vinegar with the thyme leaves and marigold flowers (p.19). Add the thyme essential oil and bottle the mixture.

Use it diluted 50:50 with water to wipe down surfaces, sinks, toilet seats and pet areas.

Lemon Zinger Floor Cleaner

Thyme & Marigold Disinfectant (p.29) forms the base of this floor cleaner, ideal for ceramic or vinyl tile floors. Do not use it on a stone floor, as vinegar can erode some types of stone, including marble.

INGREDIENTS
- 250ml/1 cup Thyme & Marigold Disinfectant (p.29)
- 750ml/3 cups distilled white vinegar
- 175ml/¾ cup lemon juice

MAKES & KEEPS
Makes enough for 4 washes. Keeps 3 months.

METHOD
Mix all the ingredients together.

Add 300ml/1¼ cups of the floor cleaner to a large bucketful (approx. 5 litres/5 quarts) of hot water from the tap. Sweep the floor and clean with a mop (no need to rinse).

Stone Floor Soap

A little linseed in this stone floor cleaner adds extra shine.

INGREDIENTS
- 250ml/1 cup Liquid Castile Soap (p.199)
- 2 tbsp linseed oil

Essential oils:
- 50 drops/½ tsp grapefruit or orange
- 50 drops/½ tsp tea tree
- 200ml/just over ¾ cup hot water

MAKES & KEEPS
Makes 450ml/just under 2 cups.
Keeps 3–6 months.

METHOD
Mix the liquid soap together with the linseed oil and essential oils. Pour the hot water over this mixture and stir gently.

To use, add 3 tbsp to a large bucket of very hot water. Clean the floor thoroughly using a mop. Rinse with clean water if desired, but not essential.

Juniper, Rosemary & Lavender Glass Cleaner

INGREDIENTS
- 250ml/1 cup distilled white vinegar

Essential oils:
- 25 drops/¼ tsp juniper
- 25 drops/¼ tsp rosemary
- 25 drops/¼ tsp lavender

MAKES & KEEPS
Makes 250ml/1 cup.
Keeps 1–2 years.

METHOD
Put the vinegar and oils in a spray bottle and shake gently. Leave for 24 hours to settle.

To use, add 2 tsp of the cleaner to 1 litre/1 quart warm water. Do not use more than this, as it will lead to streaks.

Apply the diluted cleaner to the glass using a clean cloth or spray from a bottle. Wipe the glass clean with a dry cloth.

— *Tip* —

TO AVOID STREAKS, DO NOT CLEAN WINDOWS WHEN THEY ARE WARM – EARLY MORNING OR DUSK IS THE BEST TIME.

Rosemary & Horse Chestnut Scouring Powder

Bicarbonate of soda lifts dirt off surfaces and is gently abrasive, so can be used to make a scouring powder. Adding dried and powdered herbs brings abrasive qualities to the scouring mixture. The horse chestnuts (conkers) also contain saponins, which have a detergent effect.

INGREDIENTS

- **4 dried horse chestnuts (the nuts only), ground**
- **15g/½oz dried rosemary leaves, ground**
- **430g/2 cups bicarbonate of soda**
- **300g/2½ cups gram (chickpea) flour**
- **20 drops rosemary essential oil (optional)**

MAKES & KEEPS

Makes 870g/5 cups.
Keeps 6–12 months.

METHOD

Put all the dry ingredients in a very dry jar (if damp, the bicarbonate of soda will react) with a tight-fitting lid. Shake well to mix. Sprinkle on the essential oil, if using, and mix again.

Sprinkle on to a damp cloth to clean bath rings, food deposits from the sink etc. For a cream cleaner, mix a little powder with an equal amount of water to form a paste.

— *Tip* —

USE THE ROSEMARY & HORSE CHESTNUT SCOURING POWDER TO CLEAN STAINED TEA CUPS – IT'S QUITE MIRACULOUS.

Thyme Disinfectant Scouring Powder

INGREDIENTS

- **250g/1 cup salt**
- **15 drops thyme essential oil**
- **15g/½oz dried thyme leaves, ground**
- **430g/2 cups bicarbonate of soda**

MAKES & KEEPS

Makes 700g/3¼ cups.
Keeps indefinitely.

METHOD

Spread the salt out on a plate and sprinkle thoroughly with the thyme oil. Mix all the ingredients together.

Use as for Rosemary & Horse Chestnut Scouring Powder (left).

THE RECIPES

Odour-busting Natural Drain Cleaner

The herbs and bicarbonate of soda control germs and help eliminate bad odours.

INGREDIENTS

- 15g/½oz dried thyme leaves, ground
- 15g/½oz dried rosemary leaves, ground

Essential oils:
- 50 drops/½ tsp thyme
- 50 drops/½ tsp basil
- 1kg/4 cups bicarbonate of soda

MAKES & KEEPS
Makes about 1030g/4½ cups.
Keeps at least 1 year.

METHOD
Place the thyme and rosemary with the essential oils into a jar. Mix well. Add the bicarbonate of soda, then shake and stir to mix thoroughly. Store in a dry, airtight jar.

To use, first run the hot tap for a few minutes to warm up the drain. Then slowly pour about 1 teacup or half a mug of the scouring powder down the plughole. Dribble in a little hot water to send it down the pipe. Leave the cleaner to work overnight, then rinse to clear.

Lemon Furniture Polish

As well as nourishing the wood with oil and giving a great shine, this polish smells wonderful.

INGREDIENTS

- 200ml/just over ¾ cup olive oil or linseed oil
- 20g/¾oz dried lemon balm or lemongrass (or 1 large handful of fresh)
- 120ml/½ cup lemon juice (from about 4 lemons)

MAKES & KEEPS
Makes 300ml/1¼ cups.
Keeps 6–12 months.

METHOD
Make an infused oil with the oil and herbs (p.20). Mix the infused oil with the lemon juice and bottle.

Shake well before use. Rub well into wooden furniture or floors with a soft cloth. This mixture will also nourish your hands while you polish!

Spicy Furniture Polish

INGREDIENTS
- 200ml/just over ¾ cup olive oil or linseed oil
- 2 tbsp ground mixed spice
- 100ml/just under ½ cup lemon juice, freshly squeezed or bought

MAKES & KEEPS
Makes 300ml/1¼ cups.
Keeps 6–12 months.

METHOD
Make an infused oil from the oil and mixed spice (p.20). Add the lemon juice to the mixture and bottle.

Use as for Lemon Furniture Polish (opposite).

— *Tip* —

USE SOFT COTTON OR FLANNEL CLOTHS FOR POLISHING, ONES THAT DON'T SHED THEIR FIBRES. I USE AN OLD COTTON SHEET CUT UP. MODERN MICRO-FIBRE POLISHING CLOTHS ARE ALSO GOOD.

Old-fashioned Furniture Polish

Courtesy of Teri Evans

This polish will improve your wood and should cut through residues left by spray polishes.

INGREDIENTS
- 115ml/½ cup turpentine or white spirit
- 225g/1 cup + 1 tbsp beeswax, grated or broken into small pieces
- 50 drops/½ tsp lavender essential oil

MAKES & KEEPS
Makes 340g/approx. 1½ cups.
Keeps indefinitely.

METHOD
Gently heat the turpentine and beeswax together very carefully in a double boiler or bain-marie. (Turpentine is flammable, so do not leave unattended.) When the wax is melted, pour into a jar and cool to hand hot. Add the lavender essential oil and stir.

The lavender will give off a lovely fragrance as you polish. It requires a little elbow grease, so you'll burn more calories using it!

Plant-based Wax for Raw Wood

INGREDIENTS
- 250g/1 cup beeswax, grated or broken into small pieces
- 250ml/1 cup turpentine
- 250ml/1 cup boiled linseed oil
- 100 drops/1 tsp lavender essential oil

MAKES & KEEPS
Makes 750ml/3 cups.
Keeps 2 years.

METHOD
In a double boiler or bain-marie, melt the beeswax in the turpentine, then add the oil. In order to spread the wax easily it needs to be warm, so you may need to reheat the wax before using; return it to your double boiler if necessary.

Brush it warm on to raw wood (it sinks in). Work your way away from it, and when it has dried completely (30–60 minutes), buff it up into a shine with a soft cloth. The more you buff the wood, the shinier it gets. You can add layers to increase the shine.

Metal Polish

INGREDIENTS
- 60ml/¼ cup infused vinegar of your choice (p.19)
- 4 tbsp fine clay powder or fine earth from your own garden if you have that type where you live (avoid stony or gritty soil, as this will scratch the metal).

MAKES & KEEPS
Makes 120g/½ cup.
Keeps indefinitely.

METHOD
Mix the vinegar and earth together in a bowl.

Rub the polish on your metal ornaments with a damp cloth. Wipe off with a dry soft polishing cloth and enjoy the shine. I have used this on brass, silver and gold with good effect.

— *Variation* —

THIS METAL POLISH CAN BE MADE WITH LEMON JUICE INSTEAD OF INFUSED VINEGAR IF DESIRED, BUT WILL ONLY KEEP IN THE FRIDGE FOR A WEEK.

Citrus Carpet Cleaner

INGREDIENTS
Essential oils:
- 25 drops/¼ tsp lemon
- 25 drops/¼ tsp orange
- 25 drops/¼ tsp lemongrass

- 500ml/2 cups distilled white vinegar
- Bicarbonate of soda, as required

MAKES & KEEPS
Makes 500ml/2 cups.
Keeps indefinitely.

METHOD
Add the essential oils to the vinegar and mix well. Leave for a day before use.

To treat stains, make a paste with a little of the vinegar and a small amount of bicarbonate of soda. Shake before use. Brush well into the stained area (an old toothbrush is ideal for this job). Leave it to dry, then vacuum it up.

You can also use this carpet cleaner diluted 1 part cleaner to 5 parts water in a carpet shampooing machine and 50:50 in a steam cleaner. Always check the manufacturer's instructions before using with your carpet shampooing machine or steam cleaner.

Spicy Laminate & Wooden Floor Cleaner

INGREDIENTS
- 250ml/1 cup vinegar – white or cider
- 2 cinnamon sticks, broken into pieces (or 15g/½oz ground cinnamon)
- 175ml/¾ cup surgical spirit/rubbing alcohol
- 2 tbsp Liquid Castile Soap (p.199)
- 500ml/2 cups warm water
- 50 drops/½ tsp orange essential oil

MAKES & KEEPS
Makes approx. 950ml/1 quart.
Keeps at least 1 year.

METHOD
Make an infused vinegar with the cinnamon sticks or ground cinnamon (p.19). Add the surgical spirit/rubbing alcohol, liquid soap, warm water and essential oil. Mix well and decant into a spray bottle for use.

Spray on and mop off with water.

Antibacterial Laminate & Wooden Floor Cleaner

INGREDIENTS
- 250ml/1 cup vinegar – white or cider
- 4g/⅛oz marigold petals
- 175ml/¾ cup surgical spirit/rubbing alcohol
- 2 tbsp Liquid Castile Soap (p.199)
- 500ml/2 cups warm water
- 50 drops/½ tsp thyme essential oil

MAKES & KEEPS
Makes approx. 950ml/1 quart.
Keeps at least 1 year.

METHOD
Make an infused vinegar with the marigold petals (p.19). Add the surgical spirit/rubbing alcohol, liquid soap, warm water and essential oil. Mix well.

Use as for Spicy Laminate & Wooden Floor Cleaner (left).

THE RECIPES

ROOM SPRAYS

Plant-based room sprays are widely used to freshen rooms. They play an important part in 'space-clearing' or 'energy-changing' exercises in the home. To make the sprays, put the ingredients into a 100ml/3½fl.oz spray bottle. Shake 24 times (a traditional number in feng shui) to make sure the essential oils are mixed, then spray abundantly around the room. It can be fun to add a small, specially programmed crystal to the bottle. All, bar the Fly Repellent on page 36, make 100ml/just under ½ cup and keep for up to 3 months.

All these room sprays are courtesy of Lucy Harmer.

Happy House Air Spray

A rich scent used to bring happiness and fun into a home, and help to relieve depression.

INGREDIENTS
- 100ml/just under ½ cup spring water

Essential oils:
- 12 drops basil
- 12 drops orange

Space-clearing Spray

This refreshing and clean odour is said to clear 'heavy' energy in the home.

INGREDIENTS
- 100ml/just under ½ cup spring water

Essential oils:
- 14 drops juniper
- 14 drops lavender
- 14 drops rosemary

Computer Energy Booster Spray

The effect of these clear-smelling oils increases concentration and boosts energy when you are working on a computer.

INGREDIENTS
- 100ml/just under ½ cup spring water

Essential oils:
- 8 drops lemon
- 8 drops lemongrass
- 8 drops pine

Helpful Angels Spray

Use when you are in need of divine assistance.

INGREDIENTS
- 100ml/just under ½ cup spring water

Essential oils:
- 8 drops frankincense
- 8 drops myrrh
- 8 drops sandalwood

Emotional Balancing Spray

For when life's ups and downs are getting to you.

INGREDIENTS
- 100ml/just under ½ cup spring water

Essential oils:
- 8 drops geranium
- 8 drops neroli
- 8 drops bergamot

Passion Spray

Speaks for itself!

INGREDIENTS
- 100ml/just under ½ cup spring water

Essential oils:
- 8 drops ylang ylang
- 8 drops patchouli
- 8 drops amber

Love Spray

To encourage love of all types into your life.

INGREDIENTS
- 100ml/just under ½ cup spring water

Essential oils:
- 8 drops rose
- 8 drops jasmine
- 8 drops sandalwood

Deep Sleep Spray

Zzzzzzzzz!

INGREDIENTS
- 100ml/just under ½ cup spring water

Essential oils:
- 12 drops lavender
- 6 drops chamomile
- 6 drops marjoram

Calm & Relaxation Spray

De-stress with this lovely spray.

INGREDIENTS
- 100ml/just under ½ cup spring water

Essential oils:
- 8 drops honeysuckle
- 8 drops cedar
- 8 drops vetivert

Protection Spray

These plants were traditionally used to protect the home against attacks or evil.

INGREDIENTS
- 100ml/just under ½ cup spring water

Essential oils:
- 14 drops geranium
- 14 drops sage
- 14 drops petitgrain

Prosperity Spray

This spray contains oils traditionally used to attract wealth.

INGREDIENTS
- 100ml/just under ½ cup spring water

Essential oils:
- 6 drops mint
- 6 drops cinnamon
- 9 drops vetivert
- 3 drops clove

Fly Repellent

Courtesy of Teri Evans

This is a very strong mix to spray around doors and windows to repel flies and other insects. It is not for the body.

INGREDIENTS
- 50ml/¼ cup spring water

Essential oils:
- 20 drops citronella
- 20 drops lavender

MAKES & KEEPS
Makes 50ml/¼ cup.
Keeps 3 months.

METHOD
Mix the water and essential oils together in the spray bottle.

Shake well, then spray around the window and door frames. Avoid contact with skin and eyes, as this is a strong mix.

POTPOURRI

Potpourri is a collection of dried or semi-dried herbs, flowers, woods and spices that is pleasant to the eye and gives off a lovely fragrance. Adding essential oils creates a stronger scent, and is also useful for refreshing the potpourri's fragrance.

To make any of these potpourris, mix the dried plant materials together in a beautiful bowl for display. Sprinkle the essential oils over the mix.

Each potpourri will keep well for 3–6 months. Refresh your mixture every so often with a few more drops of essential oils.

> *In our house we are devotees of Radha and Krishna (the Divine Couple of the Vedic tradition), almost every day we offer flowers on our altar to Thakurji (the Divine in statue form). I make potpourri from these special prasaadam flowers. Prasaadam means 'mercy of God'; it gives you mercy or grace in the form of spiritual blessings.*

Rainbow Potpourri

INGREDIENTS
- 2 handfuls of dried rose petals (red, pink, yellow and orange)

A few of any of the following dried flowers and leaves:
- marigolds
- lavender
- hydrangea
- forget-me-nots
- lemon balm
- rosemary
- sage

Essential oils:
- 8 drops lavender
- 8 drops lemon balm
- 8 drops geranium
- 8 drops rose or rose geranium

Winter Festivities Potpourri

Collect together enough of the following to fill your chosen display bowl:

INGREDIENTS
- holly leaves (handle with care!)
- holly berries
- cedar leaves
- ivy leaves
- small pine cones
- pine needles
- dried orange peel
- 1 tsp cloves
- 1 nutmeg, freshly ground
- glitter, to add some sparkle (optional)

Essential oils:
- 10–20 drops cinnamon
- 10–20 drops orange
- 5–10 drops pine

Breathe-easy Potpourri

This potpourri can help with breathing difficulties. Gather a mixture of the following to fill your bowl.

INGREDIENTS
- pine needles
- rosemary sprigs (broken into small pieces)
- eucalyptus leaves
- sage leaves
- bay leaves
- cedar leaves
- a few whole star anise

Essential oils:
- 10–20 drops peppermint
- 10–20 drops clary sage
- 10–20 drops pine

ECO-LAUNDRY PRODUCTS

Using eco-laundry products involves cleaning with a mixture of soap and alkaline substances (such as bicarbonate of soda and washing soda), then removing soap residues and neutralizing the alkaline with vinegar. Herbs and oils are added for aroma and antimicrobial or soothing properties.

You can buy in solid and liquid soap to use in these recipes, or make your own. Soap making is fun and rewarding, but it must be approached with care as it can be dangerous if not properly done. See page 194 for general instructions on soap making and moulds, paying special attention to the safety measures.

Travellers' Anti-bug Laundry Soap

Courtesy of Tanya Smart

This variation gives travellers extra protection from bugs and insects.

INGREDIENTS
Lye:
- 140g/5oz sodium hydroxide
- 400g/14oz water

Oil blend:
- 135g/4¾oz olive oil
- 180g/6⅓oz sunflower oil
- 620g/22oz coconut oil

Essential oils:
- 2½ tsp lavender
- 100 drops/1 tsp Virginian cedarwood
- 100 drops/1 tsp juniper
- 50 drops/½ tsp basil

MAKES & KEEPS
Makes about 12–14 average-sized bars. Keeps years if well made, though the odour of the essential oils wears off.

METHOD
Follow the instructions as for Lavender Laundry Soap (opposite), taking note of the safety measures in the general soap-making instructions (p.194).

Prepare the lye first, then heat and cool the oil blend before adding the lye to it. Add the essential oils only after you have achieved trace.

Lavender Laundry Soap

Courtesy of Tanya Smart

Handy for handwashing, stain removal and a travelling laundry solution, this soap is used grated in laundry liquid and powder recipes.

INGREDIENTS
Lye:
- 140g/5oz sodium hydroxide
- 400g/14oz water

Oil blend:
- 135g/4¾oz olive oil
- 180g/6⅓oz sunflower oil
- 620g/22oz coconut oil

Extras:
- 5 tsp lavender essential oil

MAKES & KEEPS
Makes 12–14 small bars (approx. 110g/4oz). Keeps several years.

METHOD
Take note of the safety measures in the general soap-making instructions (p.194) before preparing this recipe.

Wearing gloves and plastic goggles, make the lye by carefully pouring the sodium hydroxide crystals into the container holding the water. Leave it to cool until 27–30°C/80–86°F. Never pour water on to the lye.

Gently heat the oil blend until the coconut oil is melted and cool until 27–30°C/80–86°F.

Carefully pour the lye into the oils and stir with the spatula until you reach 'trace'; this is when the movement of the spatula creates a line on the top of the mixture – a trace that doesn't disappear. It is a sign that your soap has reached full saponification – when the lye has turned the oils to soap – and indicates your mixture is ready. To reach trace usually takes about half an hour, but soap has its own timescale! Keep stirring continuously and very thoroughly, all around the sides and the bottom of the pan.

When you've achieved a trace, add the essential oil. Ladle a little of the soap mixture into a bowl. Mix the essential oil into this small amount of soap mixture. Then mix this well into the whole batch.

Next, pour the mixture into mould(s) and cover (with a bit of board and then towels to insulate). Place the mixture out of the way for 24 hours.

After 24 hours, remove it from the mould(s), wearing gloves to protect against residual lye. Leave for another 24 hours to dry. You can then cut up the soap if you need to.

Wash all your equipment with very hot water and lots of washing-up liquid. Wear washing-up gloves (remember that the remnants will still be caustic) and rinse very thoroughly.

As with all soap, leave it to 'cure' in a well-ventilated place for 4–6 weeks. This ensures all the caustic effect of the lye has worn off.

LAUNDRY LIQUIDS

To make these laundry liquids, first stir the washing soda into a little of the hot water in a bucket until it is dissolved. Then add the bicarbonate of soda (or borax, if using; see box opposite) and stir until dissolved. Mix in the liquid soap and stir gently to avoid too much frothing up.

When all of these ingredients are dissolved, add the essential oils and the rest of the water. Stir gently, then funnel into storage bottles. If you don't have liquid soap, you can add 190–250g/¾–1 cup pure vegetable soap flakes or about half a bar of grated soap instead, dissolving it in a little boiling water before mixing in.

Shake well to remix before each use, as the ingredients will separate while standing.

For all these laundry liquids, with the exception of the Gentle Soap Nut Laundry Liquid on page 44, add ¼–⅓ cup per load of washing to the compartment or drum.

Citrus Laundry Liquid

INGREDIENTS
- 125ml–250ml/½–1 cup Liquid Castile Soap (p.199)
- 250g/1 cup washing soda
- 250g/1 cup bicarbonate of soda or borax (borax makes a stronger mix, but bicarbonate of soda is better for people with sensitive skin; see box, opposite)
- 4.5 litres/4¾ quarts hot water

Essential oils:
- 100 drops/1 tsp lemon
- 50 drops/½ tsp grapefruit

MAKES & KEEPS
Makes 4.5 litres/4¾ quarts.
Keeps at least 1 year.

Concentrated Lavender Laundry Liquid

INGREDIENTS
- 125ml–250ml/½–1 cup Liquid Castile Soap (p.199)
- 250g/1 cup washing soda
- 250g/1 cup bicarbonate of soda or borax (borax makes a stronger mix, but bicarbonate of soda is better for people with sensitive skin; see box, opposite)
- 4.5 litres/4¾ quarts hot water
- 2 tsp lavender essential oil

MAKES & KEEPS
Makes 4.5 litres/4¾ quarts.
Keeps at least 1 year.

— *Tip* —

ADD MORE LIQUID SOAP IF YOU NEED A STRONGER WASHING LIQUID. LIQUID CASTILE SOAP IS PREFERABLE, BUT IF YOU'RE UNABLE TO USE CASTILE, ANY LIQUID SOAP WILL DO.

ECO-LAUNDRY PRODUCTS

Spicy Laundry Liquid

INGREDIENTS

- 125ml–250ml/½–1 cup Liquid Castile Soap (p.199)
- 250g/1 cup washing soda
- 250g/1 cup bicarbonate of soda or borax (borax makes a stronger mix, but bicarbonate of soda is better for people with sensitive skin; see box, right)
- 4.5 litres/4¾ quarts hot water

Essential oils:
- 100 drops/1 tsp lavender
- 50 drops/½ tsp orange
- 25 drops/¼ tsp cinnamon

MAKES & KEEPS

Makes 4.5 litres/4¾ quarts.
Keeps at least 1 year.

Luxury Laundry Liquid

INGREDIENTS

- 125ml–250ml/½–1 cup Liquid Castile Soap (p.199)
- 250g/1 cup washing soda
- 250g/1 cup bicarbonate of soda or borax (borax makes a stronger mix, but bicarbonate of soda is better for people with sensitive skin; see box, right)
- 4.5 litres/4¾ quarts hot water

Essential oils:
- 100 drops/1 tsp rose geranium
- 25 drops/¼ tsp neroli
- 25 drops/¼ tsp jasmine
- 10 drops rose (optional, as expensive!)

MAKES & KEEPS

Makes 4.5 litres/4¾ quarts.
Keeps at least 1 year.

Anti-psoriasis Laundry Liquid

INGREDIENTS

- 125ml/½ cup Liquid Castile Soap (p.199)
- 250g/1 cup washing soda
- 250g/1 cup bicarbonate of soda
- 4.5 litres/4¾ quarts hot water

Essential oils:
- 100 drops/1 tsp lavender
- 50 drops/½ tsp bergamot

MAKES & KEEPS

Makes 4.5 litres/4¾ quarts.
Keeps at least 1 year.

Caution

Borax, or sodium borate, is a naturally occurring mineral salt found in dry lake beds. It is a strong cleanser and whitener, and can treat mildew. Borax contains boron, a chemical that occurs in all vegetables and fruits not grown on exhausted soil, and is important for brain, bone and immune function. However, people with delicate sensitive skin often find borax an irritant, and there is some evidence that it could be harmful to health, especially hormonal health, and the male reproductive system. Borax is no longer available in the UK, where 'borax substitutes' (sodium carbonate with soap and vinegar) are sold instead. After researching this subject I am happy to include borax in a recipe, but do research the subject yourself before making a decision. If you do use borax, as with any strong alkaloid, handle it with care; it can irritate the skin and should not be inhaled.

THE RECIPES

Gentle Soap nut Laundry Liquid

This liquid is suitable for babies and young children, wool and delicate fabrics.

INGREDIENTS
- 125ml/½ cup weak chamomile vinegar (made with 1 tsp chamomile flowers to 125ml/½ cup vinegar infused for 1 week, p.19)
- 60g/1 cup soap nuts
- 1 litre/1 quart filtered or spring water

Essential oils (optional):
- 30 drops/⅓ tsp lavender
- 30 drops/⅓ tsp chamomile

MAKES & KEEPS
Makes around 600ml/2½ cups (enough for 20 loads in a washing machine).
Keeps 6–12 months.

METHOD
Put the vinegar, soap nuts and water into a large lidded pan. Place on a medium heat and bring to a low boil. Simmer gently for 30 mins with the lid on.

Remove from heat, mash the nuts (with a potato masher) and simmer for another 30 mins, this time with the lid off to let the liquid reduce. Remove from heat.

When cool, strain the liquid and press well before adding the essential oils, if using. Store in an airtight container.

To use, add around 60ml/4 tbsp per wash to your washing machine (half this in an HE or high-efficiency machine). As with all washing liquids, you can put it in the drawer of the machine or in the drum.

Pets' Bedding Laundry Liquid

Use this to discourage fleas.

INGREDIENTS
- 250ml/1 cup Liquid Castile Soap (p.199)
- 250g/1 cup washing soda
- 250g/1 cup bicarbonate of soda or borax (borax makes a stronger mix, but bicarbonate of soda is better for people with sensitive skin; see box, p.43)
- 4.5 litres/4¾ quarts hot water

Essential oils:
- 100 drops/1 tsp lavender
- 50 drops/½ tsp tea tree

MAKES & KEEPS
Makes 4.5 litres/4¾ quarts.
Keeps at least 1 year.

METHOD
Mix gently before each use. Use 60–100ml/¼–⅓ cup per load of washing.

Space-clearer's Washing Powder

The essential oils in this recipe are used to cleanse and transform negative energy, so this powder is ideal for washing clothes before a space-clearing exercise.

INGREDIENTS
- one 100–120g/3½–4oz bar of laundry soap, grated (about 1 cup)
- 125g/½ cup washing soda
- 200g/just over ¾ cup borax, if available (see box, p.43); if not use another 125g/½ cup washing soda
- 125g/½ cup bicarbonate of soda

Essential oils:
- 50 drops/½ tsp lavender
- 50 drops/½ tsp rosemary
- 50 drops/½ tsp juniper

YOU WILL NEED
- A FOOD PROCESSOR

MAKES & KEEPS
Makes enough for 30–60 washes.
Keeps 6 months or more.

METHOD
Make using the method for Super-strong Citrus Washing Powder (right).

Use 1–2 tbsp per wash.

— *Tip* —

BEFORE YOU USE THESE LAUNDRY POWDERS, DO ONE WASH WITH JUST A HALF MUG OF PLAIN WASHING SODA. THIS WILL CLEAN OUT ANY RESIDUES FROM YOUR OLD WASHING POWDER, WHICH COULD OTHERWISE REACT WITH YOUR HOMEMADE ECO-MIX AND CAUSE A YELLOW COLOUR.

Super-strong Citrus Washing Powder

This recipe contains borax (see box, p.43), which must be handled very carefully.

INGREDIENTS
- one 100–120g/3½–4oz bar of laundry soap, grated (about 1 cup)
- 125g/½ cup washing soda
- 200g/just over ¾ cup borax, if available (see box, p.43); if not use another 125g/½ cup washing soda
- 125g/½ cup bicarbonate of soda

Essential oils:
- 50 drops/½ tsp lemon
- 50 drops/½ tsp mandarin or orange

YOU WILL NEED
- A FOOD PROCESSOR

MAKES & KEEPS
Makes enough for 30–60 washes.
Keeps 6 months or more.

METHOD
Add the essential oils to the soap, then whisk or mix in a food processor to make a finer, powdered soap.

Add the washing soda, borax and bicarbonate of soda to the food processor, and mix all the ingredients well for 3–5 minutes.

To use, add 1–2 tbsp to the powder section of your washing machine drawer.

Baby-soft Washing Powder

INGREDIENTS
- 250ml/1 cup distilled white vinegar
- 1 tsp chamomile flowers
- 1 tsp rose petals
- 1 tsp lavender flowers
- 250g/1 cup finely grated Lavender Laundry Soap (p.41) or other vegetable oil soap
- 250g/1 cup washing soda
- 250g/1 cup bicarbonate of soda

YOU WILL NEED
- A FOOD PROCESSOR

MAKES & KEEPS
Makes approx. 750g/4 cups.
Keeps indefinitely in a sealed container.

METHOD
Make an infused vinegar of chamomile, rose and lavender (p.19).

Place the grated soap in a large bowl. Stir in the washing soda and bicarbonate of soda. Gradually pour in the infused vinegar, a little at a time. This will make it foam up and thicken into a paste, so don't add too quickly.

Whisk the mixture. You can do this by hand, but a food processor will be much easier, as it needs to be very thoroughly mixed. Whisk until it becomes a powder, then leave it to stand for an hour. The mixture will appear even more powdery, just like a washing powder. Stir again and store in a sealed (airtight) container.

You will need 2–3 tbsp for each full load of washing.

Soapwort Wool Wash

INGREDIENTS
- 60g/2oz dried soapwort leaves and stems, or roots (or 120g/3 cups of fresh)
- 1 litre/1 quart water
- 250ml/1 cup distilled white vinegar (or floral vinegar as for Baby-soft Washing Powder, left)
- 20 drops lavender or lemon essential oil (optional)

YOU WILL NEED
- A FOOD PROCESSOR

MAKES & KEEPS
Makes approx. 500ml/2 cups 'soapwort tea', enough for 3–4 washes.
Keeps 12 months.

METHOD
Boil the soapwort leaves and stems in the water for approximately 10 mins (if you are using roots, boil for 20 mins) with the lid on until the mixture has reduced by one third. Leave to cool, then mix in a blender (the liquid will become frothy). Leave it for a few hours for the froth to die down, then strain well.

Add the white vinegar, or the floral vinegar if you prefer a softer scent. Mix in the essential oil, if desired.

Store in an airtight container. To use, add 120–180ml/½–¾ cup to your washing water.

Eco-powered Laundry Whitener

This fresh-smelling whitener relies on the bleaching power of lemon juice.

INGREDIENTS
- juice of 5 lemons
- 1 litre/1 quart white distilled vinegar
- 20 drops lemon essential oil

MAKES & KEEPS
Makes approx. 1 litre/1 quart (enough for about 4–8 washes).
Keeps up to 6 months.

METHOD
Mix the ingredients together.

Add 125ml/½ cup of this whitener plus 60–125g/¼–½ cup bicarbonate of soda to your regular washing liquid/powder, plus another 60–125ml/¼–½ cup in the rinse compartment.

— *Tip* —

LINE DRYING IN THE SUN IS THE BEST WAY TO KEEP CLOTHES FRESH, AND THE SUN ITSELF IS THE BEST WHITENER.

Zesty Stain-remover

The basic principle of a stain remover is to use a concentrated amount of washing product. Try using this on colour-fast clothes.

INGREDIENTS
- 4 tbsp Super-strong Citrus Washing Powder (p.45) or Baby-soft Washing Powder (opposite)
- juice of 1 lemon

MAKES & KEEPS
Makes approx. 60ml/¼ cup.
Keeps 2–3 months.

METHOD
Mix a small amount – about 1–2 tbsp – of your homemade washing powder with the lemon juice to make a paste. Then mix in the remaining washing powder. Store in a small jar.

As soon as you notice a stain, rub in a little of your stain-busting paste and put the item in the laundry basket, to await its normal wash. As with all stain removers, this remover is most effective if you treat the stain before it sets.

— *Tip* —

ANOTHER STAIN-REMOVAL METHOD IS TO SCRUB UNDILUTED LIQUID CASTILE SOAP (P.199) INTO STAINS. LEAVE FOR 30–60 MINS AND WASH AS NORMAL.

Wood Ash Detergent-free Washing Liquid

Courtesy of Marc Luyckx

Able to wash effectively in washing machines without any detergent, this is a very strong alkaline product (potash or lye). Prepare it on a tiled floor and wear gloves and goggles while working with it.

INGREDIENTS
- just over ½ bucket of sieved wood ash
- boiling water

YOU WILL NEED
- A COFFEE FILTER

MAKES & KEEPS
Makes approx. ¼ bucket.
Keeps indefinitely.

METHOD
Pour boiling water into the bucket until it reaches 4–5cm (1½–2in) above the ash. Mix it thoroughly, cover and leave to stand for 12 hours, stirring occasionally.

Stir, then filter through a muslin. Carefully dispose of the ash (it is strongly alkaline) and rinse out the cloth and bucket.

Let the liquid settle, then place a sheet of kitchen paper, folded into 4, over the hole in a funnel. Add a coffee filter and strain the liquid through this into a solid plastic container. The liquid will be yellow to light brown in colour, but this will not affect clothes in any way (note: there are no suds).

To use, put 125ml/½ cup of the washing product into the washing compartment of your machine. Add 125ml/½ cup vinegar-based fabric softener (opposite) into the washing compartment. Note: for washes on 0°–30°C/32–86°F, use half as much again of both liquid and of vinegar.

For whitening: add an equal volume of washing soda with hot water and the washing liquid to the washing compartment.

SOFT-TOUCH HERBAL FABRIC CONDITIONERS

These easy-to-make fabric conditioners use a weak infused vinegar as their base. Vinegar, an acid, basically removes all traces of soap from the fabric, making it feel soft.

All these recipes make 1 litre/1 quart (enough for about 12 washes).

Sweet & Soft Fabric Conditioner with Rose

INGREDIENTS
- 1 tbsp fragrant rose buds or petals
- 1 litre/1 quart white distilled vinegar

Essential oils:
- 50 drops/½ tsp lavender
- 25 drops/¼ tsp chamomile
- a few drops rose essential oil (optional)

KEEPS
Keeps 1–2 years.

METHOD
Infuse the roses in the vinegar (p.19). Add the essential oils to the infused vinegar.

To use, put 80ml/⅓ cup into the rinse compartment of the washing machine.

Skin-calm Fabric Softener

INGREDIENTS
- 2 tbsp marigold flowers
- 1 litre/1 quart white distilled vinegar

Essential oils:
- 50 drops/½ tsp lavender
- 50 drops/½ tsp bergamot
- a few drops rose essential oil (optional)

KEEPS
Keeps 1–2 years.

METHOD
Infuse the marigold flowers in the vinegar (p.19). Then add the essential oils to the infused vinegar.

To use, put 80ml/⅓ cup into the rinse compartment of the washing machine.

Antibacterial Fabric Softener

INGREDIENTS
- 1 litre/1 quart white distilled vinegar

Essential oils:
- 50 drops/½ tsp lavender
- 50 drops/½ tsp tea tree
- 25 drops/¼ tsp thyme

KEEPS
Keeps indefinitely.

METHOD
Mix all the ingredients together and bottle.

Use 125ml/½ cup in the rinse stage of your wash (check the manufacturer's instructions for how to do this in your machine).

Pets' Bedding Fabric Conditioner

INGREDIENTS
- 1 litre/1 quart white distilled vinegar

Essential oils:
- 50 drops/½ tsp lavender
- 50 drops/½ tsp orange
- 50 drops/½ tsp tea tree

KEEPS
Keeps indefinitely.

METHOD
Make and use as described for Antibacterial Fabric Softener (above).

HERBAL MOTH REPELLENTS

Traditional moth balls are toxic, so you might want to make your own plant-power alternatives.

To make each of the moth-repellent sachets, you will need a small piece of thin cotton cloth cut into a circle approx. 15cm (6in) in diameter, as well as silk or wool thread. Simply mix the dried herbs together in a bowl and sprinkle the essential oil, if using, over the mixture. Then lay your cloth on a flat surface and spoon half your herb mixture into the centre. Draw together the side of the cloth and fasten tightly at the top with a piece of wool or silk thread.

Each of the moth-repellent recipes makes 2 sachets, which will keep well for up to a year.

Before you pack clothes away for storing, make sure they are properly cleaned. Use a fabric conditioner as a rinse after washing. Air clothes well in the sun if you can before packing, then place these moth-repellent sachets between your folded clothes.

Lavender & Rosemary Moth Repellent

INGREDIENTS
Dried herbs:
- 2 tsp lavender flowers
- 2 tsp rosemary leaves and flowers
- 1 tsp thyme leaves
- 1 tsp cloves

Cedar & Southernwood Moth Repellent

INGREDIENTS
Dried herbs:
- 2 tsp cedar wood ground into small shavings
- 2 tsp southernwood leaves
- 1 tsp cloves
- 1 tsp thyme leaves

Essential oils (optional):
- 20 drops lavender
- 20 drops cedar wood

Moth-destroying Spray

If you already have moths, stronger methods are needed.

INGREDIENTS
- 1 litre/1 quart boiling water
- 50g/2oz dried thyme
- 20g/¾oz dried cloves
- 2 tbsp neem oil

Essential oils:
- 50 drops/½ tsp thyme
- 50 drops/½ tsp lemon

- 1 tsp Liquid Castile Soap (p.199)

MAKES & KEEPS
Makes 1 litre/1 quart.
Best used fresh, but will keep 1–2 months.

METHOD
Pour the boiling water on to the thyme and cloves. Leave to cool, then strain and add the neem oil and essential oils, plus the liquid soap. Mix thoroughly and store in a spray bottle.

If possible, put the affected clothes in the freezer for 2 days to begin the moth-killing process. Then spray them once, thoroughly, with your moth-destroying spray. Check carefully for signs of moths every week or so for a few weeks following. Repeat the process if required.

Desert-style Moth Repellent

INGREDIENTS
Dried herbs:
- 2 tsp shredded sagebrush
- 2 tsp white sage
- 1 tsp cloves
- 1 tsp southernwood

Essential oils (optional):
- 20 drops clove
- 20 drops sage

KEEPING WELL

Here you will find a range of do-it-yourself mineral and vitamin supplements, tonics and teas that can be taken every day, as well as protection and nourishment for the skin, remedies for the mind and spirit, and more…

Linseed Rehydration Tea

Being fully hydrated can make an enormous difference to how well you feel, and remain. Tea from linseeds/flax seeds is perfect for rehydrating. Rich in omega-3 fatty acids from the seeds, the tea nourishes the cell membranes, and tones and protects the digestive tract from top to bottom. This recipe gives maximum rehydration.

INGREDIENTS
- 2 tbsp linseeds/flax seeds
- 1 litre/1 quart water

MAKES & KEEPS
Makes approx. 250ml/1 cup, enough for 3 days. Keeps up to 3 days in the fridge.

METHOD
Put the seeds and water in a pan and bring to the boil. Remove from the heat and leave to stand with the lid on for 12 hours or overnight.

Next day, bring to the boil again and simmer for 1 hour. Strain the tea, reserving the seeds. These can be eaten – add to porridge or to a biscuit mix, with some sultanas.

Put 4 tablespoons of the remaining liquid into a large (ideally 1 pint/20fl.oz) mug. Dilute the thick liquid with half boiling and half cold water.

Drink 1 mug of the tea 3 times daily, half an hour before a meal.

— *Tip* —

IF YOU ARE IN A RUSH, YOU CAN MAKE LINSEED TEA THE QUICK WAY. THIS SIMPLE METHOD MAKES ENOUGH FOR ONE DAY'S TEA: BOIL 1 TBSP OF LINSEEDS/FLAX SEEDS AND 250ML/ 1 CUP WATER IN A PAN UNTIL THE WATER IS REDUCED BY HALF. DRINK ONCE OR TWICE DAILY TO SOOTHE IRRITATION. THE TEA KEEPS FOR UP TO 3 DAYS IN THE FRIDGE.

Probiotic Lemonade

Courtesy of Lynn Rawlinson

This delicious, probiotic drink can help restore the good bacteria in our digestive tract, easing bloating, irritable bowel syndrome (IBS) and trapped wind.

INGREDIENTS
- whey from one 450g/16fl.oz pot of natural organic live yogurt (see below)
- 100g/½ cup sugar
- 160g/½ cup honey
- 3.5–4 litres/3½–4 quarts freshly filtered water, to top up as required
- juice from 12 lemons

MAKES & KEEPS
Makes up to 4 litres/4 quarts.
Keeps up to 2 weeks in the fridge.

METHOD
To make the whey, place a thickish piece of muslin over a bowl and attach it with a thick rubber band or string. Pour the pot of yogurt into this and leave for 1 hour.

Scoop the yogurt back into its pot. In the bowl you will have a clearish liquid – the whey containing the probiotics or helpful bacteria.

Place the sugar and honey into a large glass jar or demijohn. Add the whey and half-fill the jar with fresh water. Add the lemon juice and top up again so that the jar is approximately three-quarters full. Put a bung or lid on. Mix the ingredients well by agitating the jar.

Keep at room temperature for 2 days; the probiotics in the whey will eat some of the sugar and multiply, leaving you with a probiotic lemonade ready to bottle.

— *Tip* —

THIS LEMONADE IS QUITE SHARP, SO YOU MAY LIKE TO SWEETEN WITH HONEY BEFORE DRINKING.

Soothing Sloe C Syrup

Courtesy of Rachel Corby

High in vitamin C, this syrup can help soothe bronchial conditions, colds, catarrh and inflammation of the throat.

INGREDIENTS
- 110g/1 cup fresh sloes (the fruit of blackthorn)
- 480ml/2 cups water
- 480g/1½ cups honey

MAKES & KEEPS
Makes approx. 700ml/3 cups.
Keeps up to 2 years in the fridge.

METHOD
Decoct the sloes in the water (p.15) for 20 mins. Do not boil. Strain and discard all the stones and plant matter.

Measure the remaining liquid. Either match what you have left with an equal volume of honey or discard any excess water so that only 360ml/1½ cups remain, then add the honey. Gently heat the liquid until all the honey has dissolved, and bottle.

Take 2 tsp 3 times a day directly from a spoon or dissolved in a herbal tea.

Do not use if pregnant or breast-feeding.

— *Tip* —

IF POSSIBLE, COLLECT THE SLOES AFTER A HARD FROST, AS THIS MAKES THEIR SKIN SOFTER AND MORE PERMEABLE. IF YOU WANT TO MAKE THE SYRUP BEFORE THE FIRST FROST, FREEZE THE SLOES BRIEFLY BEFORE USING.

Rosehip C Syrup

In Britain during the Second World War there was a shortage of fruit, so vitamin C deficiency became a concern. The Women's Institute (WI) organized mass gatherings of rosehips and produced rosehip syrup on a large scale, to a recipe provided by the Ministry of War. This recipe is based on that.

INGREDIENTS
- 200g/4 cups fresh rosehips, finely chopped
- 875ml/3½ cups boiling water
- 500 ml/2 cups cold water
- 200g/1 cup sugar

YOU WILL NEED
- DOUBLE THICKNESS MUSLIN OR JELLY BAG

MAKES & KEEPS
Makes about 500ml/17 fl.oz.
Keeps for 1 year until opened, then keep in the fridge and use within 1 month.

METHOD
Drop the freshly picked and finely chopped rosehips into the boiling water. Stir, remove from the heat and stand for 20 mins. Strain by allowing to drip through the double thickness muslin or jelly bag. Return the hips from the muslin to a pan. Wash the muslin or jelly bag immediately after – you'll need it for the next stage of the recipe.

Add the strained juice and 2 cups of cold water to the pan. Bring to the boil. Stir, remove from heat and allow to stand for 10 mins. (Doing it twice ensures you get all the vitamin C.)

Strain again through the muslin or jelly bag. Do not squeeze, but allow it to drip. This is to avoid tiny, irritating rosehip hairs getting in your preparation. As an extra precaution, pour back the first 125ml/½ cup of liquid that comes through, and make it drip through again.

Put the juice into a clean saucepan, bring to the boil, then boil with the lid off for 5 mins. Add the sugar and boil briskly for another 5 mins. Pour into small, sterilized bottles.

Pour on to puddings and cereal, drink with hot or cold water as a cordial or take 1–2 tsp up to 3 times daily to protect against colds and flu.

— *Tip* —
TO FURTHER PRESERVE SYRUPS, STERILIZE THEM AFTER BOTTLING (SEE PP.21–22).

Many Berry Cordial

Courtesy of Wizz Holland

This cordial is delicious with fizzy water or poured over ice cream or yogurt. It is rich in vitamin C, so you can also take it like a medicine, a spoonful as it is or diluted in hot water, to ward off or treat colds.

INGREDIENTS
- 110g/1 cup fresh berries (a mix of hawthorn, rosehips, elderberries, blackberries, raspberries or whatever you can find)
- 480ml/2 cups water
- juice of 1–2 lemons
- 480g/1½ cups honey

MAKES & KEEPS
Makes approx. 700ml/3 cups.
If unopened, will keep 1 year in the fridge. Once opened, drink within a few weeks.

METHOD
Make in the same way as Soothing Sloe Syrup (p.53), but add the lemon juice to each 200ml/ just over ¾ cup of liquid before adding the honey. Keep the pulp to make Many Berry Fruit Leather (p.56).

Elder, Rosehip & Rowan Berry Oxymel

This is a vitamin C-packed, immune-boosting honey and vinegar delight.

INGREDIENTS
2 handfuls of each of the following, removed from the stems:
- elderberries
- rosehips
- rowan berries
- 1 litre/1 quart Apple Cider Vinegar (p.165)
- approx. 750g/2¼ cups honey

MAKES & KEEPS
Makes about 1.2 litres/5 cups.
Keeps around 2 years.

METHOD
Make an infused vinegar with the berries (p.19).

Measure the liquid and add an equal amount of honey. Gently heat to dissolve, then bottle.

Take 1–2 teaspoons 3–4 times daily to help fight viral infections.

Many Berry Fruit Leather

Courtesy of Wizz Holland

This recipe was inspired by the lush-smelling pulp left over from making Many Berry Cordial (p.55).

INGREDIENTS

- 1kg/approx. 2–3 cups fruit pulp, left over from the Many Berry Cordial (p.55), plus what you need of apples, blackberries, rosehips etc. to make up the weight
- juice of 1 lemon
- 150g/½ cup honey

YOU WILL NEED

- FLAT BAKING TRAYS, LINED WITH GREASEPROOF PAPER
- ADDITIONAL GREASEPROOF PAPER, FOR ROLLING THE LEATHER

MAKES & KEEPS

Makes 20–30 strips.
Keeps 1–2 weeks, or up to 3 months if frozen.

METHOD

In a saucepan, gently cook the pulp with the added fruits until all are mushy. Push the pulp through a sieve to remove pips, stems and so on, then mix in the lemon juice and honey.

Spread the mixture out thinly and fairly evenly over the flat, lined trays. Leave to dry out in an oven set on the lowest temperature for 3–5 hours, or until it feels rubbery but set.

Slice into strips and make little rolls. Do this by rolling the strips together with a strip of greaseproof paper or foil, to avoid the mixture sticking to itself. Store in a big jar, ideally glass so that you can enjoy looking at the colourful collection.

— *Tip* —

YOU CAN USE ANY FRUIT TO MAKE 'LEATHER' IN A SIMILAR WAY. EXPERIMENT BY ADDING TASTY AND FRAGRANT FLOWERS, SUCH AS ROSE OR HONEYSUCKLE, OR SPICES.

Easy Iron Tonic

A very simple, easy-to-make iron and mineral tincture.

INGREDIENTS

- 200g/1 cup unsulphured (brown) dried apricots (or hunza apricots, de-stoned), roughly chopped
- 1 tbsp molasses
- 15g/½oz dried nettle tops (or 30g/1 cup fresh), roughly chopped
- 750ml/3 cups vodka

MAKES & KEEPS

Makes 700ml/3 cups. Keeps at least 2 years.

METHOD

See pp.18–19 for full instructions on how to make tinctures.

Place all the ingredients in a jar, seal and leave to brew. After 4 weeks, strain the liquid through muslin and bottle.

Take 2 tsp daily in warm water or lightly carbonated water as an iron tonic. If you are very anaemic, support your liver by taking 1 tsp 1–2 times daily of the tincture component of the Detox Complex (p.61). Easy Iron Tonic is not suitable for children under 7.

Super-green Juice

This juice is incredibly nutritious, packed with minerals, vitamins and health-giving enzymes.

INGREDIENTS

- 60g/2oz fresh wheatgrass or oatgrass

YOU WILL NEED

- A JUICER

MAKES & KEEPS

Makes 60ml/¼ cup juice.
Drink immediately.

METHOD

Put the grass through a juicer and enjoy. If you don't have a juicer, just add the grass to a smoothie.

KEEPING WELL

Vinegar Calcium Tonic

Courtesy of Jeanne Rose

An edible tincture for healthy bones, full of calcium.

INGREDIENTS
- 3 handfuls of fresh dandelion roots and leaves (dig these up yourself or buy them at a farmers' market), roughly chopped
- approx. 625ml/2⅔ cups Apple Cider Vinegar (p.165)

MAKES & KEEPS
Makes approx. 500ml/2 cups.
Keeps 1 year.

METHOD
Make an infused vinegar with the dandelion (p.19), leaving to infuse for 6 weeks. The roots will develop and exude a milky substance into the vinegar.

Strain and bottle.

Use in salad dressings and marinades or sprinkled over cooked greens. Each tbsp contains more than 175mg calcium – one-sixth of the adult recommended daily allowance.

Detoxing Mineral Vinegar

Nettles are a panacea of the plant world, used for aching joints, skin allergies or a general detoxing/cleansing. They are rich in minerals, vitamins and protein (p.241).

INGREDIENTS
- 3 handfuls of freshly picked nettle tops (or dried if you can't get fresh)
- 500ml/2 cups Apple Cider Vinegar (p.165)

MAKES & KEEPS
Makes 500ml/2 cups.
Keeps 2 years.

METHOD
Make an infused vinegar with the nettles (p.19).

Take 1–2 tbsp daily, in water or with food.

Leafu Protein Supplement

Courtesy of Michael Cole

There is a way of making 'leafu', an edible curd, from grass and stinging nettles to access the valuable protein and amino acids they contain.

INGREDIENTS
- 1kg/2lb freshly picked nettle tops (mixed with any other edible greens, including grass, if you wish)

YOU WILL NEED
- A BLENDER

MAKES & KEEPS
Makes approx. 25g/1oz leafu
(enough for 2 meals).
Keeps up to 1 week in the fridge.

METHOD
Purée the nettles in a blender, adding a small amount of water if necessary. Filter the juice through very fine cloth.

Heat the filtered juice just up to boiling point, so that a green 'froth' appears on the surface. Skim this off and put in a very fine cloth (the holes need to be tiny to retain the 'froth', which contains the protein). This 'froth' can be eaten freshly as it is or added to smoothies, soups or stews.

Alternatively, make into a curd by pressing slowly but very firmly to get all the fluid out (this may take several hours). The protein-rich curd can be cut up and added to food.

Multi-mineral Powder

Wild plants are often richer in minerals than cultivated ones. This wild herb powder can be sprinkled on to soups and stews or added to smoothies or juices for an instant health boost.

INGREDIENTS
Collect as many of the following wild herbs as you can:
- burdock root
- dandelion leaves and root
- nettle leaves and root
- plantain leaves
- ground elder leaves
- peppermint
- red clover
- thyme
- sage
- yellow dock root

Alternatively, buy a range of dried herbs.

KEEPS
1 year.

METHOD
Dry the plant material and grind to a powder in a coffee grinder. Mix thoroughly and store in an airtight container.

Take 2–3 tsp daily as a food supplement. You can add to a green smoothie or infuse in vinegar to make a multi-mineral vinegar (p.19).

Aloe Vera Nourish-all

Aloe vera contains hundreds of health-giving nutrients. To get the full benefit from this amazing miracle plant, use the leaves fresh.

INGREDIENTS
- ½ aloe vera leaf, without the green skin
- ½ cucumber, chopped
- 125ml/½ cup apple juice, freshly juiced or bought

YOU WILL NEED
- A BLENDER

MAKES & KEEPS
Makes 150ml/⅔ cup. Eat immediately.

METHOD
Cut the aloe vera leaf lengthways and scrape out the gel inside. Add the gel to the other ingredients in a blender and blend until smooth.

Drink once a week, taking a month off every 6 months. Do not take continuously without a break.

Do not use aloe vera internally during menstruation, or if you are pregnant or have liver or gall bladder problems or haemorrhoids.

Milk Vetch, Ginseng & Nettle Stress-support Tonic

INGREDIENTS
- 50g/2oz dried milk vetch root, chopped
- 50g/2oz dried ginseng root, chopped
- 50g/2oz dried Siberian ginseng root, chopped
- 1 litre/1 quart water
- 25g/1 cup chopped fresh nettle tops (or 25g/1oz dried)
- 2 tbsp quality honey (preferably manuka)
- 500ml/2 cups pure vegetable glycerine

MAKES & KEEPS
Makes 1 litre/1 quart.
Keeps 1 year.

METHOD
Decoct the roots in the water, boiling for 15 mins in a large covered pan (p.15). Add the nettles and leave to cool.

Strain and if necessary boil further to reduce it or add water to produce 500ml/2 cups of liquid. Remove from the heat and leave to cool for 10 minutes.

Add the honey and stir to dissolve. Add the glycerine and mix well, then bottle.

Take 1 tsp 2–3 times daily to boost immunity and relieve stress.

Walnut Flower Remedy for Adapting to Change

Courtesy of Lucy Harmer

Flower remedies harness flowers' energetic properties to help balance emotions. The most famous one is Dr Bach's Rescue Remedy. Following tradition, make flower remedies on a bright sunny day around 10am.

INGREDIENTS
- 3–4 stems of walnut flowers/leaves, about 15cm/6in in length (gather mainly female flowers; see box, below).
- 500ml/2 cups water
- approx. 250ml/1 cup brandy (more if required)

MAKES & KEEPS
Makes approx. 500ml/2 cups.
Keeps 2 years.

METHOD
Put the flowers and leaves in a saucepan with the water. Bring to the boil and simmer for about 30 mins without a lid, stirring constantly. Remove from heat, add the lid and leave to cool.

Strain into a glass bottle. Mix with an equal amount of brandy.

Keep in a dark place and fill a dropper bottle when you wish to use.

Take 3–5 drops 3 times a day or when you are feeling stressed.

> *Female walnut flowers are small, green and fig-shaped, while the male flowers are fat green catkins.*

THE RECIPES

Weight Loss Spice

A spice mix of plants that help to burn fat.

INGREDIENTS
Dried herbs:
25g/1oz ground ginger
- 25g/1oz ground cardamom
- 25g/1oz ground turmeric
- 5 tsp cayenne pepper

MAKES & KEEPS
Makes approx. 80g/3oz.
Keeps 1 year.

METHOD
Mix the spices together well.

Drink as a tea, using 1 tsp of spice per mug of boiling water (p.15).

Drink 2–3 times daily.

Weight Loss Tea

These herbs can help to calm the appetite and speed metabolism without making you jumpy. Use alongside a healthy diet and also consider a detox programme.

INGREDIENTS
- 50g/2oz green tea
- 25g/1oz fennel seeds
- 25g/1oz dried dandelion leaves

MAKES & KEEPS
Makes 100g/4oz.
Keeps at least 1 year.

METHOD
Mix the ingredients together well. Make the tea using 1 tsp per mug (p.15).

Drink 2–4 mugs daily.

— *Variation* —

ALTERNATIVELY, MAKE A SOLID SPREAD. TO DO THIS, MELT A 340G/12OZ JAR OF EXTRA-VIRGIN COCONUT OIL BY PLACING THE JAR INTO A BOWL OF HOT WATER. ONCE MELTED, MIX THE SPICES IN THOROUGHLY. ALLOW TO SET. TAKE 1 TSP 2–3 TIMES DAILY, EITHER DIRECTLY OFF THE SPOON OR ADDED TO FOOD. (EVEN THOUGH IT IS AN OIL, COCONUT OIL SPEEDS METABOLISM AND HELPS THE BODY TO BURN OFF FAT.)

Detox Complex

Courtesy of Louise Idoux

In this mixture, the herbs encourage the liver to clear toxins into the bile. The prune juice takes them out of the body through bowel movements.

INGREDIENTS
Tinctures (either bought or homemade, pp.18–19) of the following:
- 30ml/2 tbsp milk thistle seeds
- 20ml/4 tsp dandelion root
- 25ml/5 tsp burdock root
- 25ml/5 tsp artichoke leaves

- 100ml/just under ½ cup prune juice

MAKES & KEEPS
Makes 200ml/just over ¾ cup.
Keeps up to 2 years.

METHOD
Mix the ingredients together and bottle.

Take 2 tsp in a little water 3 times daily.

Do not give detoxing medicines to children under 12.

Detox Tea

This makes a mixture of dried herbs from which to make a daily tea.

INGREDIENTS
Dried herbs:
- 15g/½oz nettle tops
- 15g/½oz dandelion leaves
- 15g/½oz ginger root, roughly ground
- 15g/½oz dandelion root, roughly ground
- 15g/½oz burdock root, roughly ground
- 2 cinnamon sticks, roughly ground

MAKES & KEEPS
Makes 100g/3½oz.
Keeps 1 year.

METHOD
Mix the ingredients and store in a jar.

Make tea using 1 tsp per mug of boiling water. Allow to infuse for 5–10 minutes (p.15).

Drink 1–3 mugs daily, adding fresh lemon juice, and honey to taste.

Do not give detoxing medicines to children under 12. Detoxing of any kind is not recommended during pregnancy or breast-feeding. If you have any health problems, you should only undertake detoxing with the guidance of a qualified healthcare practitioner.

Mineral-rich Seaweed Bath

To nourish the skin, encourage detoxification, relieve muscle and joint stiffness, and help the circulation.

INGREDIENTS
- 25g/1oz dried kelp
- 25g/1oz dried dulse

MAKES
Makes enough for 1 bath.

METHOD
It works best to put dried seaweed into a muslin bag, otherwise it blocks your drain and is difficult to clean up. If you can gather fresh seaweed, put a couple of handfuls of each into your bath while running.

Soak in as hot a bath as is comfortable for around 30 mins.

The Big Cleanser Smoothie

Courtesy of Neil McNulty

INGREDIENTS
- 1 apple
- 2 small bananas
- 2 handfuls of mixed fresh or frozen berries
- juice of 1 lemon (no pips)
- 10 fresh rosemary leaves (no stems)
- Herbal tea: 1 small mug with peppermint (1 tsp or 1 tea bag) and nettle (2 tsp or 2 tea bags), infused for 5–10 mins

YOU WILL NEED
- A BLENDER

MAKES & KEEPS
Makes 1–2 servings.
Drink immediately.

METHOD
Blend all the ingredients together and drink right away.

Warm the Bones Smoothie

Courtesy of Neil McNulty

Ideal for people who feel the cold, or for treating rheumatism.

INGREDIENTS
- 2.5cm/1in piece fresh ginger root
- ½ tsp ground cinnamon
- 1 tsp ground turmeric
- 3 tbsp coconut milk (or organic live natural yogurt)
- 2 large bananas
- 2 pears
- Herbal tea: 1 small mug of chamomile tea (made from 1 tsp dried chamomile or 1 tea bag infused for 5–10 minutes).

YOU WILL NEED
- A BLENDER

MAKES & KEEPS
Makes 1–2 servings. Drink immediately.

METHOD
Blend all the ingredients together and drink right away.

Winter Warmer Tea

INGREDIENTS
- 20g/¾oz dried ginger root
- 2 cinnamon sticks
- 20g/¾oz dried liquorice root

MAKES & KEEPS
Makes 60g/2oz herb mixture.
Keeps 1 year.

METHOD
Loosely grind the ginger, cinnamon and liquorice in a coffee grinder – you don't need a fine powder. Store in a jar.

Make tea using 1 tsp per mug infused for 5–10 minutes (p.15). Take 1–3 times daily to improve circulation.

Kidney-strengthening Tea

A daily drink to support the kidneys.

INGREDIENTS
- 20g/¾oz dried cornsilk
- 20g/¾oz dried nettle leaves

MAKES & KEEPS
Makes 40g/1½oz herb mixture.
Keeps up to 1 year.

METHOD
Mix the herbs together. Make tea using 1 tbsp to a teapot of boiling water.

Drink over the day.

Cornsilk is the dried stamens of corn on the cob — if you pick fresh or buy with the outer leaves still on, you see these long, thin pale yellow/green strands all around the cob. Remove these and lay to dry on a flat tray in a warm, dark place. When dry they look like brown hair. Break them up and mix with the nettles.

Chilblain Oil

Courtesy of Sue Wine

INGREDIENTS
- 1 tbsp vegetable oil (any, but almond and sesame work well)

Essential oils:
- 5 drops geranium
- 1 drop lavender
- 1 drop rosemary

MAKES & KEEPS
Makes 1 tbsp for 1 application.
Use immediately.

METHOD
Mix the oils together and rub into chilblains when they are sore.

Equinox Tea for the Changing Seasons

Courtesy of Christine Herren-Valette

This tea helps to prepare for the important transition from winter to spring, and summer to autumn — key times when people fall ill, as the body tries to go through a powerful detoxification process.

INGREDIENTS

Dried herbs:
- 12g/4 tbsp nettle tops
- 7g/3 tbsp downy birch leaves
- 5g/2 tbsp marigold flowers
- 3g/3 tsp blackcurrant leaves
- 3g/3 tsp meadowsweet flowers

MAKES & KEEPS
Makes 30g/1oz herb mixture.
Keeps up to 1 year.

METHOD
Mix the herbs together and make a tea using 1 tsp per mug of boiling water (p.15).

Take 2–3 times daily.

Honey, Lemon & Ginger for Colds

Courtesy of Sue Wine

INGREDIENTS
- 2.5cm/1in piece fresh ginger root
- 2 tsp honey
- juice of ½ lemon

MAKES & KEEPS
1 mug.
Drink immediately.

METHOD
Peel and slice the ginger thinly. Place in a mug of boiling water, then add the other ingredients. Leave to brew for 5–10 mins, then drink (you can also eat the bits of ginger). It will make you sweat and banish your head cold.

Hyssop Cough Syrup

Courtesy of Teri Evans

INGREDIENTS
- 225g/¾ cup + 2 tbsp honey
- 60ml/¼ cup hot water
- 2 tbsp dried hyssop, moistened with 1 tbsp hot water
- 1 tsp aniseed, crushed

MAKES & KEEPS
Makes approx. 250ml/8½fl.oz.
Keeps up to 1 year in the fridge until opened.

METHOD
Heat the honey and water gently in a saucepan until syrupy. Then leave to simmer for 5 mins, regularly skimming off any scum that forms.

Next, add the hyssop and aniseed. Stir, cover and simmer for 30 mins. Remove the lid and leave to cool slightly before straining into a jar.

Adults: Take 1 tbsp up to 6 times daily.

Children: Take 1 tbsp up to 4 times daily.

Turmeric Honey Antibiotic

To help your body fight any infection

INGREDIENTS
- 1 jar of runny honey
- 1 jar the same size of ground turmeric

KEEPS
2 years.

METHOD
Empty both jars into a bowl and mix thoroughly. Return the mixture to the original jars. Handle turmeric carefully, as it can stain.

Adults: Take 1 tsp 3–4 times daily.

Children: Take ½ tsp 3 times daily.

Birch Aromatic Syrup for Coughs & Sore Throats

Courtesy of Johanna Herzog

INGREDIENTS
- 500ml/2 cups vodka
- 2 handfuls of fresh birch leaves or leaves and buds
- 400g/2 cups sugar (white or brown)

MAKES & KEEPS
Makes approx. 750ml/26fl.oz.
Keeps indefinitely.

METHOD
Mix all the ingredients together in a saucepan and let them simmer gently for approx. 5 mins. Strain and bottle while the syrup is still hot.

Adults: Take 1–2 tsp every 4 hours.

Thyme & Liquorice Cough Syrup

Courtesy of Joe Nasr

INGREDIENTS
- 50g/2oz dried liquorice root, chopped
- 1.4 litres/6 cups hot water
- 20g/¾oz dried rubbed thyme leaf
- white or brown sugar, variable amount
- 35ml/2 tbsp + 1 tsp pure vegetable glycerine

MAKES & KEEPS
Makes approx. 1 litre/34fl.oz.
Keeps at least 1 year.

METHOD
In a saucepan, soak the liquorice root in the hot water for 1 hour. Cover with a lid, switch on the heat and simmer for 25 mins.

Turn off the heat. Mix in the thyme leaf and allow to cool.

Strain the liquid through muslin and measure the liquid's exact weight. Stir an equal amount of the sugar thoroughly into the liquid.

Heat the mixture gently to around body temperature – lukewarm – and stir at this heat until the sugar is dissolved. Then mix in the glycerine and remove from the heat. Pour into bottles and seal when cooled.

Adults: Take 1–3 tsp 2–3 times daily after meals.

Children: Take ½–1 tsp 2–3 times daily after meals.

Garlic & Echinacea Infection-busting Tincture

Growing your own echinacea if you can is a very good idea, since it is particularly effective as a fresh tincture and is very expensive to buy.

INGREDIENTS
- 30g/1oz dried echinacea root, or 60g/⅔ cup fresh roots and tops, chopped
- 2 heads garlic, peeled and crushed
- 500ml/2 cups vodka

MAKES & KEEPS
Makes almost 500ml/2 cups.
Keeps 2 years.

METHOD
Place all the ingredients in a large lidded jar. Make a tincture (pp.18–19).

Adults: Take 1 tsp 3–5 times daily for acute infections.

Children (under 12): Take 10–20 drops in a little cooled boiled water.

Anti-viral Elder

Courtesy of ChaNan Bonser

An alcohol-free tincture. Use to prevent any viral infection or to aid recovery.

INGREDIENTS
- 6–8 heads fresh elderflowers
- 500ml/2 cups pure vegetable glycerine
- juice of 2 lemons
- 6–8 heads fresh elderberries

MAKES & KEEPS
Makes approx. 500ml/2 cups.
Keeps 1 year.

METHOD
Pick the elderflowers off the heads and put straight into a bowl. Cover the flowers with the glycerine, ensuring they are completely covered. Add the lemon juice.

Put into a jar. Leave for at least 1 month, shaking at least once a day, while you wait for the elderberries to ripen. When the elderberries are ripe, remove the berries from the stems and place the berries into a jar. Separately, strain the elderflower mixture through a sieve and pour this liquid over the elderberries, ensuring they are all covered. Stir well and mash the mixture. Leave for at least 1 further month, shaking every day.

After this time, strain the liquid again through muslin, and rebottle.

Take 1 tsp as required, either as it is or diluted in your favourite drink.

— *Tip* —
PICK YOUR ELDERFLOWERS ON A DRY DAY, IDEALLY AFTER ANY DEW HAS BEEN BURNT OFF.

Barrier Bar for Busy Hands

Courtesy of Annie Powell

Protects hardworking hands from dry skin.

INGREDIENTS
- 160ml /²⁄₃ cup virgin olive oil
- 100g/²⁄₃ cup beeswax, grated
- 25 drops lavender or chamomile essential oil (or a mix of the two)

YOU WILL NEED:
- PATTY TINS
- GREASEPROOF AND BROWN PAPER

MAKES & KEEPS
Makes 4–6 bars.
Keeps at least 1 year.

METHOD
In a double boiler or bain-marie, gently melt the olive oil and beeswax over a low heat. Mix together thoroughly.

Remove from heat and add the essential oil(s). Pour into patty tins and leave to cool. Turn out and wrap in greaseproof paper, then brown paper.

Elderberry Oxymel

This remedy is an excellent vitamin C tonic and anti-viral. Good for all ages, except for babies under one year of age as it contains honey, it can also help arthritis and rheumatic problems. It tastes lovely with hot water and also makes a refreshing drink when made with sparkling water.

INGREDIENTS

- 7–8 heads fresh elderberries
- 750ml/3 cups Apple Cider Vinegar (p.165)
- 700g/2½ cups unpasteurized honey

MAKES & KEEPS

Makes approx. 1 litre/1 quart.
Keeps 1–2 years until opened, then keep in the fridge and use within 6 months.

METHOD

Gather the elderberries when they are ripe. Use to make an infused vinegar (p.19).

Pour the liquid into a saucepan and heat gently. Add the honey and stir it until it dissolves, taking the pan off the heat after 2 mins. Do not boil, as this would destroy some of the honey's powerful properties. Pour into bottles.

Take 1 tsp daily to prevent colds and flu.
To treat them, take 1 tsp 3–4 times daily.

Elders' Sherry Tonic

This tonic is a tincture to help older bodies to stay healthy and strong. There is a variation for women and men using different types of ginseng.

INGREDIENTS

- 25g/1oz dried milk vetch root
- 20g/¾oz dried nettle tops
- 25g/1oz dried ginkgo
- 100g/½ cup unsulphured (brown) dried apricots, chopped
- 750ml/3 cups of your favourite sherry
- for men: 25g/1oz dried ginseng root or Panex (American) ginseng
- for women: 25g/1oz dried Siberian ginseng root
- 100ml/6 tbsp + 2 tsp hawthorn tincture (bought-in or Mother of the Heart Tincture, p.75)
- 200ml/¾ cup + 5 tsp elderberry syrup or Anti-viral Elder (opposite)

MAKES & KEEPS

Makes approx. 1 litre/1 quart.
Keeps 2 years.

METHOD

Grind the roots to a rough powder in a coffee grinder and place in a jar. Add the nettles, ginkgo, ginseng and apricots, and cover with the sherry.

Leave in a cool, dark place for 3 weeks, turning daily. Strain well and add the hawthorn tincture and elderberry syrup before bottling.

Take 1–2 tbsp in a little water daily.

Elders' Alcohol-free Tonic

INGREDIENTS
- 1 litre/1 quart water
- 25g/1oz dried milk vetch root
- 20g/¾oz dried nettle leaf
- 25g/1oz dried gingko
- for men: 25g/1oz dried ginseng root or Panax (American) ginseng
- for women: 25g/1oz dried Siberian ginseng root
- 100g/½ cup unsulphured (brown) dried apricots, chopped
- 340g/12oz jar of honey
- 185ml/¾ cup Hawthorn Flower Syrup (p.157)
- 185ml/¾ cup elderberry syrup (p.20) or Anti-viral Elder (p.66)

MAKES & KEEPS
Makes 1 litre/1 quart. Keeps 1 year until opened, then in the fridge for 1 month.

METHOD
Decoct the herbs and apricots in the water, boiling for 10 minutes (p.15). Leave to cool, strain and press, then simmer the liquid for 10–15 minutes to reduce it to 600ml/2½ cups.

Add the honey and continue to gently heat for 2–3 minutes, stirring to dissolve the honey, then mix in the Hawthorn Flower Syrup and add the elderberry syrup or Anti-viral Elder. Bottle into 5 or more small bottles.

Take 1–2 tbsp daily in water.

Brain-booster

There is some evidence that these ingredients are beneficial to the brain and could help prevent dementia.

INGREDIENTS
- 340g/12oz jar of extra virgin coconut oil
- 30g/1oz dried ground rosemary
- 50g/2oz dried ground gingko

MAKES & KEEPS
Makes 420g/15oz.
Keeps up to 1 year.

METHOD
Stand the jar of coconut oil in a bowl of warm water to melt it.

Mix the rosemary and gingko together in a bowl, then pour the melted coconut oil over the mixture. Stir well and pour into jars.

Take 2–3 tsp twice daily for maximum effect.

Coconut Inflammation Beater

Ginger and turmeric have been shown to have powerful anti-inflammatory properties, helping to prevent and cure many degenerative diseases. Coconut oil also has healing properties, reducing inflammation, improving metabolism and nourishing the brain. It makes a pleasant and easy way to take the spices.

INGREDIENTS
- 340g/12oz jar of extra virgin coconut oil
- 100g/4oz ground turmeric
- 50g/2oz ground ginger

MAKES & KEEPS
Makes 490g/18oz.
Keeps up to 1 year.

METHOD
Melt the coconut oil in a double boiler or bain-marie. Mix the turmeric and ginger in well and pour into jars.

Take 2 tsp twice daily.

Bedsore & Blister Preventative

Rub this surgical spirit tincture into the skin to toughen it and to help prevent bedsores and blisters.

INGREDIENTS
- 10–15 fresh marigold flowers
- 1 small bunch of fresh sage leaves
- 1 small bunch of fresh lavender, stripped from stems
- 1 small bunch of fresh thyme, stripped from stems
- 1 litre/1 quart surgical spirit/rubbing alcohol

MAKES & KEEPS
Makes 1 litre/1 quart.
Keeps indefinitely.

METHOD
Make a tincture from the herbs and surgical spirit or rubbing alcohol (pp.18–19).

Rub into any areas of skin that need toughening, 2–3 times daily.

— *Tip* —

THE ACT OF GENTLY RUBBING THE SKIN IMPROVES CIRCULATION AND SO HELPS PREVENT BEDSORES. FOR DELICATE SKIN, APPLY A HEALING OINTMENT OR CREAM FREQUENTLY.

WELL-BEING TEAS

A great way of enhancing your well-being is to get into the habit of drinking herbal teas daily.

The following recipes are for dried herb mixtures that can be made into teas.

All dried herb mixtures should be stored in airtight jars away from the light – they'll keep at their best for up to a year this way.

To make the tea, mix 1–2 tsp of the dried herb mixture into a mug of boiling water and leave to infuse (p.15). Once teas are made, they should be consumed immediately for best results.

Sleepy Tea

This tea will calm a wide-awake mind.

INGREDIENTS
- 20g/¾oz passion flower
- 60g/2oz valerian
- 20g/¾oz lemon balm
- 15g/½oz lavender

MAKES
Makes 115g/4oz herb mixture.

METHOD
Drink a mug of sleepy tea half an hour before bed every night.

Anti-stress Tea

INGREDIENTS
- 20g/¾oz lemon balm
- 20g/¾oz wood betony
- 20g/¾oz oatstraw
- 20g/¾oz skullcap
- 20g/¾oz vervain
- 8g/¼oz lavender

MAKES
Makes 108g/4oz herb mixture.

METHOD
Drink 1–3 mugs daily, with honey to sweeten if required.

Cheering Tea

Courtesy of Dedj Leibbrandt

This colourful tea will bring a smile to your face.

INGREDIENTS
- 15g/½oz lavender flowers
- 8g/¼oz cornflowers
- 8g/¼oz marigold petals
- 15g/½oz lime flowers
- 15g/½oz sage
- 2 tsp dill seeds
- 1 tsp poppy seeds

MAKES
Makes 65g/2¼oz herb mixture.

METHOD
Drink 2–4 mugs daily.

Grief Tea

The cure for grief is to mourn — to allow feelings to surface, acknowledge them, let tears flow and wash away the grief. This is a tea to help that process happen in a gentle way.

INGREDIENTS
- 15g/½oz lemon balm
- 15g/½oz rosebuds or petals
- 15g/½oz heather flowering tops

MAKES
Makes 45g/1½oz herb mixture.

METHOD
Drink 3–5 mugs daily.

Pregnancy Tea

Take this tea during the last 3 months of pregnancy to strengthen and tone the womb, and your mind and heart, in preparation for birth.

INGREDIENTS
- 50g/2oz raspberry leaves
- 50g/2oz rosebuds

MAKES
Makes 100g/4oz herb mixture.

METHOD
Drink 1–2 mugs daily.

In the last 3 weeks of pregnancy, add 50g/2oz lady's mantle to the mix.

Continue to take the tea daily for at least 1 month after the baby is born to help the womb return to its normal size and recover its tone.

Quick Wake Up

Get going without caffeine!

INGREDIENTS
- 1 mug of rosemary tea (made by infusing 1 tsp dried rosemary in 1 mug of boiling water for 10 mins, then straining)
- ½ tsp cayenne pepper

MAKES
Makes 1 mug. Drink immediately.

METHOD
Stir the cayenne pepper into the warm rosemary tea and drink. You're off!

Oak Bud Remedy for Strength

If you have never tried 'tree hugging', start now! Lean right into the oak to connect with its deep strength and power of endurance, as you ask the tree to lend you its strength.

INGREDIENTS
- about 100 oak buds
- 250ml/1 cup brandy

MAKES & KEEPS
Makes 250ml/1 cup. Keeps for 2 years.

METHOD
Make a tincture with the oak buds and brandy (pp.18–19).

Decant the strained tincture into a small dropper bottle and take 1 drop any time extra courage and strength is needed.

THE RECIPES

MASSAGE OILS

Massage is a very powerful tool for keeping well. 'Rubbing' was considered a vital part of a physician's work in Europe before the Dark Ages, when much useful medical knowledge was lost, and it is still integral to Chinese medicine and Ayurveda. The following recipes blend various oils for healing massage. They can be used as oils, or made into a soft balm with a little beeswax for a no-spill version.

Oils or balms should be stored in airtight containers away from the light, and will keep for up to a few months, depending on how long the base oil keeps (see infused oils, page 20).

To use, put a little of the oil or balm into your hands and massage into skin.

Stimulating Massage Oil

This is good for warming and stimulating muscles, joints and skin.

INGREDIENTS
- 75ml/⅓ cup almond oil infused with rosemary leaves, dried or fresh (p.20)
- 2 tbsp mustard seed oil

Essential oils:
- 5 drops rosemary
- 5 drops black pepper
- 5 drops cardamom
- 5 drops ginger

MAKES & KEEPS
Makes 75ml/⅓ cup.
Keeps 1–2 months.

METHOD
Mix the ingredients in a bottle and gently shake.

Relaxing Massage Oil

INGREDIENTS
- 120ml/½ cup Lavender-infused Oil (opposite)

Essential oils:
- 10 drops lavender
- 10 drops clary sage

MAKES & KEEPS
Makes 120ml/½ cup.
Keeps 1–2 months.

METHOD
Mix the ingredients in a bottle and gently shake.

— *Variation* —

FOR A SENSUAL MASSAGE BALM, USE 125ML/½ CUP OF ROSE AND JASMINE INFUSED OIL (P.20) AND 10 DROPS EACH OF JASMINE, SANDALWOOD, ROSE AND YLANG YLANG ESSENTIAL OILS.

Stress-busting Massage Balm

INGREDIENTS
- 125 ml/½ cup Lavender-infused Oil (right)
- 1½ tsp grated beeswax

Essential oils:
- 10 drops lavender
- 10 drops sandalwood
- 10 drops cedarwood
- 10 drops bergamot

MAKES & KEEPS
Makes 130ml/½ cup.
Keeps around 3 months.

METHOD
Melt the beeswax into the infused oil in a double boiler or bain-marie. Add the essential oils and pour into a container.

Lavender-infused Oil

Lavender is a relaxing and soothing herb with anti-inflammatory properties.

INGREDIENTS
- 30g/1oz dried lavender flowers
- 180ml/¾ cup olive oil
- 180ml/¾ cup grapeseed oil

MAKES & KEEPS
Makes approx. 350ml/1½ cups.
Keeps around 6 months.

METHOD
Fill a jar with the best, most fragrant lavender flowers you can find. Cover with the olive and grapeseed oils. Leave to infuse for 3–4 weeks. Strain well and bottle.

Birch Massage Oil

Courtesy of Johanna Herzog

Soothing, for inflamed skin and cellulitis.

INGREDIENTS
- 750ml/3 cups oil or a mixture of oils of your choice (apricot kernel, macadamia, jojoba, pure almond oil or coconut are some of my favourites)
- 2 handfuls of fresh birch leaves, chopped
- 3 tbsp vodka
- grated zest of 1 lemon

MAKES & KEEPS
Makes approx. 750ml/3 cups.
Keeps 6–12 months.

METHOD
Put the ingredients into a jar. Leave in a warm place for 3 weeks, then strain through muslin and bottle the liquid. Shake well before use.

Fiery Muscle Rub

A deep heat rub for aches and pains.

INGREDIENTS
- 250ml/1 cup Fire Cider (p.165)
- 250ml/1 cup Hot Oil (p.155)

MAKES & KEEPS
Makes 500ml/2 cups. Keeps at least 12 months.

METHOD
Mix the ingredients together in a bottle. Shake before each use.

> **Caution**
> Wash your hands well after applying the Fiery Muscle Rub, as getting it in your eyes or anywhere delicate would really smart.

Stretch Mark Prevention Oil for Pregnant Women

Massage this oil into the abdomen and breasts before bedtime every day from the start of the second trimester. For the third trimester, also apply it in the morning.

INGREDIENTS
- 2 tbsp Heal-all Marigold Oil (p.81)
- 2 tbsp Comfrey Oil (p.80)
- 5 tsp rosehip oil
- 2 tsp evening primrose oil
- 1 tsp vitamin E oil (or another 1 tsp evening primrose oil)

Essential oils:
- 10 drops mandarin
- 10 drops lavender

MAKES & KEEPS
Makes 100ml/just under ½ cup.
Keeps 6 months.

METHOD
Blend the oils in a bottle and use as much as required, as instructed above.

Mother of the Heart Tincture

Hawthorn, known in herbal medicine as 'the mother of the heart', is used to support the heart and circulation for pretty much any condition. This is a simple tincture, with the added advantage of tasting good.

INGREDIENTS
- 2 large handfuls of fresh hawthorn berries (dried if you can't find fresh)
- 750ml–1 litre/3–4 cups vodka

MAKES & KEEPS
Makes 700–900ml/3–3¾ cups.
Keeps at least 2 years.

METHOD
Make a tincture with the berries and vodka (pp.18–19).

Take 1 tsp in water daily to help protect against heart disease.

Always consult a qualified health professional for advice if you have a heart condition.

Clear Vision Drops

Courtesy of Sensory Solutions

Although these drops can be used to treat and prevent eye problems, they also have an effect on the 'energetic' vision — our ability to see solutions and directions in life.

INGREDIENTS
Tinctures (pp.18–19):
- 30ml/2 tbsp bilberry tincture
- 30ml/2 tbsp heather tincture

MAKES & KEEPS
Makes 60ml/¼ cup.
Keeps 2 years.

METHOD
Mix the tinctures in a dropper bottle ready to take.

Take a few drops of the mixture 4 times daily. If you wish, repeat an affirmation 3 times out loud as you do so. The affirmation should be related to what you want from the drops (for example, 'I can see a clear path to the solution I seek'). It will thus connect you to their purpose every time you take them.

Agrimony Teachers' Gargle

Perfect for easing and restoring overworked throats.

INGREDIENTS
- 1 litre/1 quart boiling water
- 30g/1oz dried agrimony
- 15g/½oz dried sage, chopped

MAKES & KEEPS
Makes approx. 950ml/4 cups.
Keeps 4 days in the fridge.

METHOD
Pour boiling water on the herbs and leave until cold. Strain and press through a muslin-lined funnel. Store the liquid in a bottle.

To use, dilute ½ mug with a little hot water. Gargle 3 times daily.

Marsh mallow Cough Syrup

Courtesy of Teri Evans

INGREDIENTS
- 1 tbsp chopped dried marsh mallow root or leaves
- 450ml/just under 2 cups water
- 340g/1¾ cups brown sugar
- 4 tbsp orange juice or juice of 1 lemon

MAKES & KEEPS
Makes about 500ml/17fl.oz.
Keeps 1 year unopened; once opened, keeps 1–2 months in the fridge.

METHOD
Soak the marsh mallow in the water overnight. Strain in the morning, then simmer the liquid with the sugar for 5 mins to make a thick syrup. Add the juice and bottle.

Take 1–2 tsp as needed.

Quick Onion Cough Syrup

Courtesy of Lucy Wells

This syrup can help to soothe a cough and fight infection in the lungs.

INGREDIENTS
- 1–2 tbsp brown sugar
- 1 onion

MAKES & KEEPS
Makes a small, variable amount – about 10 tsp.
Use over 2–3 days.

METHOD
Put the sugar on a small plate or a saucer. Cut the onion and put on to the sugar, cut sides down.

Leave for 24 hours. The sugar pulls out the onion's juices and together they make the syrup in the saucer.

Take 1 tsp every 1–2 hours until the cough is soothed.

— *Tip* —
ACCORDING TO ONION LORE, A CUT ONION IN A ROOM WILL REMOVE ANY UNWANTED INFECTION/IMPURITY FROM THE AIR (THOUGH IT IS NOT RECOMMENDED FOR USE IN FOOD PREPARATIONS!). PUTTING CUT ONION IN A SOCK AND HOLDING IT TO THE EAR CAN HELP GREATLY WITH EARACHE.

Ear Oil

Courtesy of Monika Ghent

Use this oil for earaches or to soften up ear wax so that it can be gently removed.

INGREDIENTS
- 2 tsp coconut oil
- 2 tsp jojoba oil

Infused oils (p.20):
- 2 tsp marigold
- 2 tsp St John's wort
- 2 tsp mullein flower

- oil from 3 x 400 IU vitamin E oil capsules

MAKES & KEEPS
Makes approx. 50ml/¼ cup.
Keeps 3–6 months.

METHOD
Gently melt the coconut oil, then mix with all the ingredients into a dropper bottle.

Shake the mixture well before using. Put 1–2 drops into each ear and close off the ear with cotton wool. Leave in overnight, removing the cotton wool the next morning.

Mullein Pile Ointment

An old effective gardener's treatment for piles was bruising a fresh mullein leaf and putting it in your underpants. Mullein leaves are velvety soft, so this is probably quite nice — on the other hand, you may prefer this recipe!

INGREDIENTS
- 20g/¾oz dried mullein leaves, or several fresh leaves, shredded
- 500ml/2 cups olive oil
- 4 tbsp grated beeswax

MAKES & KEEPS
Makes approx. 500g/2 cups.
Keeps up to 1 year.

METHOD
Make an infused oil by gently heating the mullein in the olive oil (p.20).

Gently heat the beeswax and the infused oil together in a double boiler or bain-marie until the wax has melted, then pour into jars. Place the lids on loosely and tighten when the mixture has cooled.

To use, wash carefully after each bowel movement and apply ointment. Can be applied 3–4 times daily in addition.

— *Tip* —

ANY INFUSED OIL CAN BE MADE INTO AN OINTMENT USING THE METHOD ABOVE.

FIRST-AID PLANT POWER

Nature's kingdom is abundant in all sorts of powerful remedies for injuries, emergencies and life's ups and downs. This chapter is packed with home remedies for soothing and healing cuts, bruises, breaks and strains, and for treating everyday ailments like colds and flu, headaches, hayfever and tummy upsets.

Antiseptic Mist

Courtesy of Louise Idoux

INGREDIENTS
- 40ml/2 tbs + 2 tsp lavender aromatic water (p.15)
- 40ml/2 tbs + 2 tsp bay aromatic water (p.15)
- 10ml/2 tsp myrrh tincture (see box below and pp.18–19)
- 10ml/2 tsp calendula tincture (pp.18–19)
- ½ tsp raw honey (preferably manuka)
- 1 drop tea tree essential oil

MAKES & KEEPS
Makes 100ml/just under ½ cup.
Keeps up to 18 months.

METHOD
Mix together in a spray bottle or mister.

Spray once or twice directly on to wounds, twice daily.

— *Tip* —

YOU CAN MAKE YOUR OWN TINCTURES BY FOLLOWING THE GUIDELINES ON PP.18–19. YOU CAN USE VODKA TO MAKE ALL TINCTURES, EXCEPT FOR TINCTURE OF MYRRH, WHICH IS MADE FROM MYRRH RESIN AND REQUIRES 90 PER CENT ALCOHOL – YOU CAN GET EVERCLEAR GRAIN ALCOHOL THAT IS 90 PER CENT FOR THIS PURPOSE.

Honey & Marigold Graze Remedy

Try this instead of painfully picking gravel out of a graze. Honey is antiseptic, with strong healing properties; combined with the amazing marigold, it makes for miraculous healing.

INGREDIENTS
- 20 or so fresh marigold flowers (or 10g/⅓oz dried)
- 340g/12oz jar of runny honey

MAKES & KEEPS
Makes 340g/12oz.
Keeps 1–2 years or more.

METHOD
Put the marigold flowers into a jar. Pour the honey over them, up to the top. Leave it for 2–3 weeks, or until you need it (there is no need to take the flowers out of the honey).

To use, slather the honey all over the grazed area. Cover with a large sticking plaster and leave overnight. The next day, carefully peel off the plaster. The honey will have pulled out all the tiny stones, leaving the wound clean.

Quick Chamomile Eye Poultice for Sore Eyes

INGREDIENTS
- 1–2 chamomile tea bags
- 2 tbs boiling water

MAKES & KEEPS
This makes enough for one or both eyes. For immediate use.

METHOD
Place the tea bags in a small bowl and cover with the boiling water. When cooled to just warm, lightly drain the bags.

Lie down and place the bags over closed eyes for 5–15 mins.

Antibacterial Honey

This do-it-yourself antibiotic is very powerful. It can be taken for any infection, especially one of the ears, nose, throat, lungs and teeth.

INGREDIENTS
- 2 heads garlic, peeled and crushed
- 60g/1 cup fresh thyme leaves and flowers, removed from stems (or rubbed if using dried)
- up to 340g/12oz jar of runny honey

MAKES & KEEPS
Makes 340g/12oz.
Keeps at least 3–6 months.

METHOD
Mix the garlic and thyme in an empty 340g/12oz jar. Pour the honey over the mixture, making sure all is covered.

Adults: Take 1 tsp 3–4 times daily.

Children: Take ½ tsp 3 times daily.

Ulcer-healing Honey

INGREDIENTS
Dried ground herbs:
- 30g/1oz liquorice root
- 30g/1oz myrrh resin
- 30g/1oz marigold flowers
- 80g/¼ cup raw honey (preferably manuka)

MAKES & KEEPS
Makes 170g/1¼ cups.
Keeps for years.

METHOD
Mix all the ingredients thoroughly and store in a jar. Apply frequently to mouth ulcers and other open sores that are not healing well.

Take 1 tsp 2–3 times daily for ulcers in the digestive system.

Spray for Strained or Sore Throats

INGREDIENTS
- 2 drops thyme essential oil
- ½ tsp pure vegetable glycerine
- 10ml/2 tsp sage tincture (pp.18–19)
- 10ml/2 tsp echinacea tincture (pp.18–19)
- 1 tbs elderberry, rowan or rosehip syrup, or a mixture (p.21)
- 4 tsp boiled water

MAKES & KEEPS
Makes 2 x 30ml/1fl.oz spray bottles.
Keeps 3–6 months.

METHOD
Beat the thyme essential oil into the glycerine. Slowly add the sage tincture, echinacea tincture, syrup and the boiled water, beating as you pour. Mix well, then bottle in small spray bottles for ease of use.

To use, spray directly into the back of the mouth as often as required.

Simple Turnip Cough Syrup

Courtesy of Anne Chiotis

An expectorant to help your lungs clear themselves of mucus.

INGREDIENTS
- 1 fresh turnip
- plenty of brown sugar

MAKES & KEEPS
Makes a variable amount.
Best used fresh, but keeps up to 2–3 weeks in the fridge.

METHOD
Hollow out the centre of a turnip, leaving 3–4cm(1¼–1½in) of flesh around the edge. Fill it with brown sugar and leave for 12 hours. A delectable syrup will form as the sugar draws the juice out of the turnip. You can simply store the turnip in the fridge, using it as your 'cup', or else decant the syrup into a jar.

Take 1–3 tsp 3 times daily.

Comfrey Oil

This makes a powerful healing oil. Dried comfrey leaves work best; fresh ones are juicy and hold too much water to use in an oil.

INGREDIENTS
- 50g/2oz dried comfrey leaves
- 500ml/2 cups olive oil or other vegetable oil

MAKES & KEEPS
Makes 450ml/just under 2 cups.
Keeps 3–12 months.

METHOD
Make as described for the Heal-all Marigold Oil (opposite).

Use in creams, ointments and liniments for healing connective tissue.

Intensive Skin Repair Balm

Courtesy of Iain Stewart

This solid, waxy balm for cracked skin, especially on hands and heels, is popular with climbers.

INGREDIENTS
- 8 tsp grated beeswax
- 2 tbs jojoba oil
- 7 tbs grapeseed oil
- 1 tbs Comfrey Oil (left)

Essential oils:
- 24 drops tangerine
- 12 drops petitgrain
- 6 drops patchouli
- 6 drops black pepper
- 6 drops cypress
- 6 drops benzoin
- oil from 3 x 400 IU vitamin E capsules

YOU WILL NEED
- 6 x 30G/1OZ SILICONE MOULDS

MAKES & KEEPS
Makes 6 blocks of 30g/1oz blocks.
Keeps for years.

METHOD
Place the beeswax, jojoba, grapeseed and Comfrey Oil in a double boiler or bain-marie. Heat for a couple of minutes until the wax has melted.

Allow to cool for 5 minutes, stirring from time to time. Then add the essential oils and vitamin E, mixing well.

Put the mixture into silicone moulds and leave overnight. It will set very hard. Remove from the moulds and store.

— *Tip* —
USE OLIVE OIL TO MAKE A
LONGER-LASTING OIL; OTHER OILS
KEEP LESS LONG.

FIRST-AID PLANT POWER

Heal-all Marigold Oil

Marigold, often known by its Latin name **Calendula***, has many excellent healing qualities and is beautifully easy to grow. Its infused oil is used alone or in many healing and nourishing balms, ointments and creams. This recipe uses the hot method, double infused.*

INGREDIENTS

- 100g/4 cups marigold flowers, freshly picked (or 30g/1oz dried)
- 450ml/just under 2 cups olive oil or other vegetable oil

MAKES & KEEPS

Makes approx. 400ml/1⅔ cups.
Keeps 3–12 months.

METHOD

Place half the marigolds in a double boiler. Heat gently in the oil. Keep on a very low heat, just warming the oil really, for 3 hours.

Remove from heat and leave to cool. When cool, strain and press through a sieve or funnel lined with muslin. Compost the remainder of the herbs.

Add the remaining marigolds to the infused oil. Repeat the simmering process for a further 2 hours, then leave to cool and strain again. This is now a double-infused oil (p.20).

Heal-all Marigold Cream

Use this cream made from pot marigolds for its antibacterial and soothing effects.

INGREDIENTS

Oil fraction:
- 100ml/6 tbs + 2 tsp Heal-all Marigold Oil (left)
- 50g/½ cup emulsifying wax

Water fraction:
- 200ml/¾ cup + 5 tsp strong marigold tea (p.15)
- 100ml/6 tbs + 2 tsp marigold tincture (pp.18–19)

Extras:
- 2ml/½ tsp benzoin tincture (Friar's Balsam)

MAKES & KEEPS

Makes 450g/just under 2 cups.
Keeps 6–12 months in the fridge.

METHOD

Make the cream following the method for Comfrey Cream for Speedy Healing (p.82).

— *Variation* —

FOR A MULTIPURPOSE ANTISEPTIC CREAM, STIR IN 3ML/½ TSP LAVENDER ESSENTIAL OIL RIGHT AT THE END OF THE PROCESS.

Comfrey Cream for Speedy Healing

Courtesy of Dedj Leibbrandt

Read the cream-making instructions (pp. 20–21) before you start. Creams made using emulsifying wax are usually foolproof.

INGREDIENTS

Oil fraction:
- 100ml/6 tbs + 2 tsp Comfrey Oil (p.80)
- 50g/½ cup emulsifying wax

Water fraction:
- 200ml/¾ cup + 5 tsp strong comfrey tea (p.15)
- 100ml/6 tbs + 2 tsp comfrey tincture (pp.18–19)

Extras:
- 2ml/½ tsp benzoin tincture (Friar's Balsam)

MAKES & KEEPS
Makes 450g/just under 2 cups.
Keeps 6–12 months in the fridge.

METHOD

Gently heat the oil fraction in a double boiler or bain-marie. Once the wax has melted, add the tea. Keep the mixture on the heat if it needs to remelt.

Next, add the water fraction and then put the pan in a basin of cold water to quickly cool it – this is called a 'cold water bath'. Whisk the mixture constantly until it emulsifies, which takes 3–4 minutes with a hand whisk. Then mix in the benzoin tincture (to preserve the cream) and pour into jars.

Apply liberally to any injury where the skin remains unbroken.

— Variation —

THE COMFREY CREAM RECIPE CAN BE ADAPTED TO MAKE ANY CREAM, SUBSTITUTING DIFFERENT HERBS TO SUIT DIFFERENT PURPOSES. YOU CAN ALSO ADD ESSENTIAL OILS FOR THEIR HEALING QUALITIES (UP TO 3ML/½ TSP EACH) WHEN YOU ADD THE BENZOIN. SEE THE 'HEAL-ALL MARIGOLD CREAM' FOR EXAMPLE (P.81), AND THE 'STOP ITCH CREAM' (BELOW).

Stop Itch Cream

Courtesy of Dedj Leibbrandt

INGREDIENTS

Oil fraction:
- 50ml/3 tbs + 1 tsp chickweed infused oil (made using 60ml/¼ cup olive oil infused with 2 tbs chickweed)
- 25g/¼ cup emulsifying wax

Water fraction:
- 100ml/6 tbs + 2 tsp strong chickweed infusion (p.15)
- 50ml/3 tbs + 1 tsp chickweed tincture (pp.18–19)
- 30 drops peppermint essential oil
- 20 drops benzoin tincture (Friar's Balsam)

MAKES & KEEPS
Makes 225g/8oz.
Keeps 1 year.

METHOD

Make in the same way as Comfrey Cream for Speedy Healing (left), stirring in the peppermint oil with the benzoin tincture.

Apply liberally to ease itching as often as needed. Do not use on broken skin.

St John's Wort Oil

This beautiful red infused oil with anti-inflammatory, healing and anti-viral action uses the sun's power to capture the healing properties of St John's wort. You have to make this oil from freshly picked flowers, and it requires sunlight to develop properly.

INGREDIENTS
- any size jar full of freshly picked St John's wort flowers
- olive oil, for covering

MAKES & KEEPS
Keeps 6–12 months.

METHOD
Pour the olive oil over your freshly picked flowers, right up to the top of jar.

Add the lid and place the jar in a sunny spot, turning daily. It takes 2–8 weeks to be ready, depending on how much sun it receives. You know it is ready because the oil goes deep red.

Strain, press and wring out through a muslin-lined sieve or funnel into a dark-coloured bottle. Compost the spent flowers.

Add more flowers and continue for a double infusion if desired, as for Heal-all Marigold Oil (p.81).

This oil is brilliant for applying to herpes and shingles, and added to any anti-inflammatory cream, ointment, liniment or rub.

Antiseptic Healing Lotion

INGREDIENTS
Tinctures (pp.18–19):
- 60ml/¼ cup St John's wort
- 60ml/¼ cup marigold

MAKES & KEEPS
Makes 120ml/½ cup.
Keeps 1–2 years.

METHOD
Mix the tinctures together.

Apply neat to bites and stings, cuts, grazes, spots, cold sores and so on.

Dilute a few drops in a mug of water to wash infected skin 2–3 times daily.

Aloe Vera Instant Burn Remedy

Aloe vera is easy to grow. Its long leaves are full of a transparent gel that can be applied directly to burnt skin, with immediate soothing and healing results.

INGREDIENTS
- 1 fresh aloe vera leaf

MAKES & KEEPS
Makes enough for 1 application.
Use immediately.

METHOD
Cut the leaf lengthways with a sharp knife.

Scrape out the gel and apply it straight to a burn.

— *Tip* —

LAVENDER ESSENTIAL OIL CAN ALSO BE APPLIED UNDILUTED TO EVEN SEVERE BURNS WITH EXCELLENT EFFECT.

THE RECIPES

Sage & Daisy Poultice for Bruises & Swellings

INGREDIENTS
- fresh sage leaves
- fresh daisies
- vinegar to cover

MAKES & KEEPS
Makes 1 application.
Use immediately.

METHOD
Gather enough herbs to cover the area. Gently heat the herbs and the vinegar together for about 5 mins. Do not boil.

Lay the herbs, still hot, out on a thin piece of cloth. Fold the cloth to a size big enough to cover the bruised area. Place it on the body, while the herbs are still hot but not in danger of burning. Wrap it with a towel to retain the heat.

Replace 1–2 times daily, as needed.

— *Variation* —

USE A VINEGAR INFUSED WITH SAGE, ROSEMARY OR COMFREY (P.19) AS A VARIATION ON THE ABOVE.

Poultice for Broken Bones & Strains

Fresh comfrey root is a miraculous healer. Keep some in the freezer so that you have it to hand whenever you need it.

INGREDIENTS
- fresh comfrey root
- approx. 3 tbs hot water

YOU WILL NEED
- A BLENDER
- GAUZE AND MICROPORE TAPE

MAKES & KEEPS
Makes 1 application.
Fresh roots keep 2 weeks in the fridge. Keeps 3–6 months in the freezer.

METHOD
Put enough comfrey root to cover the affected area in a blender, with the hot water to help it whizz up. Mix to a smooth paste. If you don't have a blender, you can grate the roots.

Apply to the affected area. Cover with gauze and micropore tape to hold the poultice in place.

It will become a hard, dry cast after a few days. At this point remove the poultice, replacing it with a fresh application.

Do not use on open wounds.

Ribwort Poultice for Infected Wounds

Courtesy of Eliot Cowan

A simple and highly effective cure.

INGREDIENTS
- fresh ribwort plantain leaves

MAKES & KEEPS
Makes 1 application.
Use immediately.

METHOD
Mash up the leaves (or chew them) to make a poultice.

Put the poultice on infected or suppurating wounds, and insect bites/stings. Change frequently.

— *Tip* —
YOU CAN USE DRIED LEAVES FOR POULTICES – JUST ADD A BIT OF HOT WATER TO MAKE IT JUICY.

Mouth Ulcer Cure

Courtesy of Eliot Cowan

An incredibly efficacious and fast-acting cure for mouth ulcers in the mouth.

INGREDIENTS
- small piece of golden thread root

KEEPS
Use immediately.

METHOD
Place a small amount of the golden root between the gums or teeth and the sore. It is very bitter, but keep sucking on it until the bitterness almost disappears, then remove.

Repeat until the ulcer is cured.

Daisy Bruise Ointment

You can use arnica instead of daisies.

INGREDIENTS
- 30–40 common daisy flowers
- 140ml/⅓ cup olive oil
- 1 tbs grated beeswax

MAKES & KEEPS
Makes 120g/4oz.
Keeps 6–12 months.

METHOD
Make an infused oil with the daisies (p.20); you should end up with 120ml/½ cup of infused oil.

Gently heat the beeswax and the infused oil together until melted. Pour into jars.

Apply to bruises 3–6 times daily or as needed.

Jewellweed Salve for Skin Infections

Courtesy of Eliot Cowan

Jewellweed is not only a good remedy against fungal skin infections, such as athlete's foot, ringworm, pityriasis versicolor and so on, but it is also an antidote to poison ivy when applied to the skin.

INGREDIENTS
- 1 handful of fresh jewellweed leaves, stems and flowers
- 250ml/1 cup olive oil
- 25g/1oz grated beeswax

MAKES & KEEPS
Makes 250ml/1 cup.
Keeps at least 1 year.

METHOD
Gently heat the jewellweed and olive oil to make an infused oil (p.20). The liquid will turn bright orange, the colour of the flowers.

Strain the mixture. Then, gently heat the beeswax into the oil to make a salve.

Apply liberally and frequently to infected skin.

— *Tip* —

YOU CAN ALSO MAKE A TEA (P.15) FROM THE JEWELLWEED AND DAB THE COOLED LIQUID ON THE INFECTED AREA FREQUENTLY.

Mullein Flower Oil for Earache

You can make this oil using either the cold- or heat-infused method — see page 20.

INGREDIENTS
- 390ml/13fl.oz jar of mullein flowers, freshly picked
- 200ml/just over ¾ cup olive oil

MAKES & KEEPS
Makes approx. 190ml/just over ¾ cup.
Keeps 3–6 months.

METHOD
Make an infused oil with the mullein flowers and olive oil (p.20). Once ready, store the bulk in a jar and a small amount in a dropper bottle for ease of administering the oil.

Put a few drops directly in the ear 3–6 times daily.

— *Variation* —

ADD 2–4ML/½–⅔ TSP OF LAVENDER ESSENTIAL OIL, WHICH IS GOOD FOR TREATING AND PREVENTING INFECTIONS.

Cold & Flu Tea

This classic remedy helps to prevent a cold if you catch it early, as you begin to shiver and feel its onset. It stimulates the circulation and promotes sweating.

INGREDIENTS
Dried herbs:
- 30g/1oz elderflowers
- 30g/1oz peppermint leaves
- 30g/1oz yarrow flowers

MAKES & KEEPS
Makes 90g/3oz herb mixture.
Keeps 1 year.

METHOD
Mix the ingredients thoroughly. Make tea (p.15) using 2–3 tsp per mug of boiling water, infused for 5 mins.

Drink freely.

— *Tip* —

MAKE ICE POPS WITH THIS TEA: MAKE UP 500ML/2 CUPS COLD & FLU TEA AND SWEETEN WITH HONEY TO TASTE. LEAVE TO COOL, THEN FREEZE IN ICE-LOLLY OR ICE-CUBE MOULDS. SUCK ON THEM TO CALM SORE THROATS AND FEVERS.

Basil Snifterchief

Courtesy of Sue Wine

A surprisingly effective remedy to protect against, and treat, sore throats and viral colds.

INGREDIENTS
- 5 drops basil essential oil

MAKES & KEEPS
Makes 1 application.
Use the same day.

METHOD
Drop the basil oil on to a handkerchief. Keep it in your pocket or under your pillow and sniff often. Just smell the oil – do not touch the handkerchief to your skin.

Xmas Survival Tummy Tonic

Helps to settle the stomach after over-indulging in rich foods.

INGREDIENTS
Dried ground herbs:
- 15g/½oz angelica root
- 15g/½oz chamomile
- 15g/½oz liquorice
- 15g/½oz marsh mallow root
- 15g/½oz artichoke roots or milk thistle seeds

- 340g/12oz jar of runny honey (optional)

MAKES & KEEPS
Makes 415g/14½oz.
Keeps 1 year.

METHOD
Mix the ground herbs thoroughly with the honey to make a paste or thick syrup.

Take 1–2 tsp in a glass or cup of hot water 1–3 times daily for as long as needed.

Headache Powders

A preventative for chronic, regular headache and migraines.

INGREDIENTS
Dried ground herbs:
- 30g/1oz ginkgo
- 15g/½oz feverfew leaves
- 30g/1oz valerian root
- 15g/½oz ginger root

MAKES & KEEPS
Makes 90g/3oz herb mixture. Keeps 1 year.

METHOD
Simply mix all the herbs together and store in a jar.

Take 1 tsp in hot water 2–3 times daily as a headache preventative.

> **Caution**
> Dehydration is a common cause of headaches, and magnesium deficiency can be a factor in migraines. If you suffer from regular headaches or migraines, consult a herbalist for tailor-made treatment.

Herbal Aspirin

Aspirin was first found in willow bark. It has been used for centuries as a painkiller for headaches and other pains, and to bring down fevers.

INGREDIENTS
Dried ground herbs:
- 60g/2oz willow bark
- 30g/1oz lavender
- 60g/2oz valerian
- 30g/1oz skullcap

MAKES & KEEPS
Makes 180g/6oz herb mixture. Keeps 1 year.

METHOD
Mix the herbs together well.

Take 1–2 tsp of the powder in a mug of water up to 4 times daily.

Homage to Hildegard Hangover Cure

Courtesy of Teri Evans

This hangover cure is based on a medieval recipe by Hildegard of Bingen. It draws upon herbs used at that time for 'swimmings of the head', 'biliousness' and so forth.

INGREDIENTS
Tinctures (pp.18–19):
- 25ml/5 tsp chamomile
- 20ml/4 tsp holy thistle
- 20ml/4 tsp milk thistle
- 15ml/1 tbs meadowsweet
- 15ml/1 tbs wood betony
- 2ml/½ tsp ginger

MAKES & KEEPS
Makes approx. 100ml/just under ½ cup. Keeps 2 years.

METHOD
Mix the tinctures together and store.

Take 1 tsp. twice before midday, dissolved in 600ml/2½ cups water.

Homemade Tiger Balm

Courtesy of Catherine Johnson

A famous pungent painkiller, originally from Burma. Apply a small amount to the temples to ease headaches or rub on to itching insect bites or tired muscles.

INGREDIENTS
- 100ml/just under ½ cup hemp oil
- 1 tbs grated or small pieces beeswax

Essential oils:
- 100 drops/1 tsp peppermint
- 60 drops/½ tsp camphor oil
- 80 drops/⅔ tsp wintergreen
- 60 drops/ ½ tsp lavender
- 60 drops/½ tsp eucalyptus

MAKES & KEEPS
Makes 120ml/½ cup.
Keeps 6–12 months.

METHOD
Gently melt the hemp oil and beeswax in a double boiler or bain-marie. Allow to cool for 5 mins, then add the essential oils.

Stir well and pour the balm into a jar.

Keep it away from eyes.

Hayfever Mead

If you can, start taking herbal hayfever medicine a week or two before you usually start to feel the allergy. Ideally, make the mead from fresh herbs, otherwise dried will do.

INGREDIENTS
- 1 handful of elderflowers
- 1 handful of thyme leaves and flowers
- 1 handful of eyebright, leaves and flowers
- 1 handful of plantain leaves
- 1 handful of chamomile flowers
- 1 handful of nettle tops
- 600ml/2½ cups mead

MAKES & KEEPS
Makes 575ml/2⅓ cups.
Keeps over 1 year.

METHOD
Gather the herbs, if using fresh.

Remove from stems, then cut up or shred.

Mix the herbs together and make a tincture using the mead (pp.18–19).

If already suffering from hayfever, take 1–2 tsp 3 times daily. To prevent onset, try ½–1 tsp.

Children can take 10–20 drops 3 times daily.

FIRST-AID KIT FOR TRAVELLERS

For travelling, it is always good to take your own remedies with you, as you may not be able to easily source some herbs while you are away. Remember that if you are flying, there will be restrictions on taking liquids and pastes in your hand luggage.

Travel Sickness Sweets

Read the sweet-making section (pp.21–22) before attempting this recipe.

INGREDIENTS
- 1 handful of fresh chopped ginger root
- 400ml/1⅔ cups water
- 300g/1½ cups brown sugar
- 30g/2 tbs butter or almond oil

MAKES & KEEPS
Makes about 20–40 sweets.
Keeps 3–4 weeks.

METHOD
Boil the ginger in the water for 20 mins. Strain and measure. If necessary, reduce the liquid further by simmering with the lid off. You're aiming for about 200ml/just over ¾ cup.

With the liquid still over the heat, add the sugar and boil until you reach 'hard-ball' stage (p.22). Remove from the heat and stir in the butter or oil.

High-Flier Sweets for Anxious Fliers

Read the sweet-making section (pp.21–22) before attempting this recipe.

INGREDIENTS
Dried herbs:
- 30g/1oz valerian root
- 15g/½oz passion flower
- 30g/1oz red clover (mildly blood thinning)
- 500ml/2 cups water
- 400g/2 cups sugar

MAKES & KEEPS
Makes 40–70 sweets.
Keeps 3–4 weeks in an airtight container.

METHOD
Boil the valerian, passion flower and red clover in the water for 15 mins. Strain, and reduce the liquid to 250ml/1 cup by simmering if necessary. Add the sugar to the liquid and boil until you reach 'hard-ball' stage (p.22).

Blood Thinning Mix for Long-haul Travellers

INGREDIENTS
- 120ml/½ cup Apple Cider Vinegar (p.165)
- 2 tbs finely chopped fresh ginger root
- 1 head garlic, cloves separated, peeled and crushed
- 2 tbs ground turmeric
- 3 tsp cayenne powder

MAKES & KEEPS
Makes 120ml/½ cup. Keeps 1–2 years.

METHOD
Make an infused vinegar using all the ingredients (p.19).

Add 1 tbsp. to a large tomato juice at the start of your flight, repeating every 3 hours.

Do not use if you are on warfarin or other blood-thinning drugs.

FIRST-AID PLANT POWER

Antiseptic Hand Sanitizer

For times when you cannot wash your hands or want to give them an extra hygiene zap.

INGREDIENTS
- 4 tbs water, boiled or distilled
- 2 tsp aloe vera gel
- 2 tbs distilled witch hazel

Essential oils:
- 15 drops lavender
- 15 drops tea tree
- 7 drops thyme

- oil from 2 x 400 IU vitamin E capsules (optional)

MAKES & KEEPS
Makes approx. 100ml/just under ½ cup. Keeps 1 month.

METHOD
Mix all the ingredients together. Decant the liquid into a pocket-sized spray bottle to use.

Spray directly on to hands only. Rub all over as if washing them.

Air-con Shield

This will help prevent you from picking up your fellow passengers' bugs.

INGREDIENTS
Essential oils:
- 50 drops/½ tsp thyme
- 100 drops/1 tsp tea tree
- 100 drops/1 tsp lavender

MAKES & KEEPS
Makes 12.5ml/2½ tsp. Keeps at least 2 years.

METHOD
Mix the essential oils together.

Sprinkle a few drops on to a tissue or cotton wool. Wipe around the air vent above your seat (and the neighbouring seats if you can) in the plane.

Mosi Spray

Courtesy of Dedj Leibbrandt

One mosi spray may work for one person but not another because of the way the herbs and oils mix with our own scent to create a new smell.

INGREDIENTS
- 150ml/⅔ cup distilled witch hazel
- 100ml/6 tbs + 2 tsp mugwort tincture (pp.18–19)

Essential oils:
- 17 drops lavender
- 17 drops thyme
- 17 drops peppermint
- 35 drops lemongrass
- 15 drops citronella

- 1 tsp emulsifier (optional)

MAKES & KEEPS
Makes 250ml/1 cup. Keeps 2 years.

METHOD
Simply mix the ingredients together and decant into a spray bottle. If you choose not to use an emulsifier, just shake well before each use.

Shake well before use. Apply to the skin as needed to deter mosquitoes.

Biting Insect Repellent

Courtesy of Michael Vertolli

This will deter mosquitoes, black flies, deer flies, horse flies, fleas and ticks. For ants, spray it for a few days at the point where they are entering the house. You can spray it on pets' bedding, but not directly on to pets.

INGREDIENTS
- 52.5ml/3 tbs + 1½ tsp water
- 42.5ml/2 tbs + 1½ tsp vodka
- 5ml/1 tsp pure vegetable glycerine

Essential oils:
- 10 drops sweet basil
- 10 drops catnip
- 10 drops lavender
- 10 drops fir
- 10 drops pine
- 10 drops citronella
- 10 drops lemon or lemongrass
- 5 drops cedar
- 5 drops patchouli

MAKES & KEEPS
Makes 103ml/just under ½ cup.
Keeps indefinitely.

METHOD
Mix all the ingredients together well and store in a spray bottle for ease of use.

Shake well before use. Spray on exposed areas, then spread the repellent around with your hands to make sure the entire surface of your skin is coated. Avoid contact with your eyes – to apply to face, spray your hands and rub it in carefully. If it gets into your eyes, rinse well with water.

Re-apply as needed; it will last for several hours.

Bug-busting Mix for Holiday Tums

Take this herbal remedy alongside natural organic live yogurt (or a probiotic capsule of 'friendly bacteria') to help protect you from 'holiday tummy'.

Please note that this recipe is NOT a substitute for eating and drinking sensibly – in certain countries, that means being very careful about water and food.

INGREDIENTS
Dried ground herbs:
- 4 tbs fennel or cardamom
- 3 tbs bayberry root
- 3 tbs cinnamon powder
- 2 tbs cloves

- 10 drops thyme essential oil
- 200ml/just over ¾ cup Apple Cider Vinegar (p.165)
- 3 tbs runny honey

MAKES & KEEPS
Makes 300ml/1¼ cups.
Keeps 6–12 months.

METHOD
Mix all the ingredients together well and put into a strong, wide-mouthed plastic bottle for travelling. Shake or stir before use.

Take 2 tsp daily in a little water, mixed with the freshly squeezed juice of ½ lemon if desired.

— Tip —

IF YOU FEEL YOU HAVE EATEN OR DRUNK SOMETHING UNWISELY, TAKE AN EXTRA DOSE OF THE BUG-BUSTING MIX THAT DAY AND THE FOLLOWING DAY.

'Lemon Sherbet' Rehydration Remedy

It's important to drink water frequently throughout the day while you're travelling, especially in hotter climes. If you feel dehydrated, this simple recipe can help replenish your body's fluids.

INGREDIENTS
- 1 litre/1 quart boiled water
- 8 tsp sugar
- 1 tsp salt
- grated zest and juice of 1 lemon

MAKES & KEEPS
Makes 1 litre/1 quart. Drink within 2 days.

METHOD
Dissolve the sugar and salt in the water. Add the lemon. Sip frequently over 1–2 days to replace fluids lost by diarrhoea, vomiting or fever.

Diarrhoea Stopper

Always consult a qualified healthcare practitioner if symptoms persist or are very severe, especially in young children who can get dehydrated very quickly.

INGREDIENTS
Dried herbs:
- 3 tsp green tea
- 3 tsp agrimony
- 2 tsp bayberry (or yellow root)
- 2 tsp oak bark
- 2 tsp ground cinnamon

MAKES & KEEPS
Makes 20g/¾oz herb mixture (enough for 4 doses).
Keeps 1 year.

METHOD
Grind the herbs to powder. Mix well and store in an airtight container.

Make the tea, using 3 tsp. mixture per mug of boiling water. Leave to cool and drink ½ tea cup up to 6 times in a day.

Anti-malaria Mix

I carry this mix with me whenever I'm travelling to a malaria area because these herbs can help protect against this serious disease.

INGREDIENTS
Tinctures (pp.18–19):
- 120ml/½ cup sweet wormwood
- 60ml/¼ cup bayberry

MAKES & KEEPS
Makes 180ml/¾ cup.
Keeps 2 years.

METHOD
Simply mix the tinctures together in a bottle and store.

Take 1 tsp 3 times daily if you are in an area where malaria is known to be active. Continue to take the mixture 1 tsp 3 times daily for 1–2 weeks after you leave the danger area.

Caution

Malaria is a potentially life-threatening illness and precautions should always be taken when travelling to countries where it is prevalent. Always consult a health practitioner and research the subject thoroughly before travelling.

Allopathic physicians recommend taking a course of drugs to prevent malaria, though most herbalists will opt for natural alternatives. While it's possible to take both drugs and herbal treatments together, it's essential you check with your health practitioner before doing so. It's also important to note that no drug or herb regime offers guaranteed protection against malaria. Always be vigilant against mosquitoes. Cover up and use nets and repellents as your first line of defence.

KITCHEN PHARMACY

Herbalism is a holistic form of healing that recognizes the close and vital links between body, mind and spirit. All three elements need to be kept in harmony and balance, as all are essential to our well-being. Spirit is the most difficult concept for many Westerners; the best explanation I've heard is from plant spirit medicine expert Eliot Cowan, which I described in my book *Holistic Anatomy* (2010):

'If you think of all the movements your body makes in an hour, then compare that to where your mind goes in the same time, you can see that the mind is way faster than the body … the mind is simply too fast for the body to grasp. Well, your spirit is to your mind what your mind is to your body — so far beyond the mind that the mind can only now and then get a glimpse of it. Yet many of us have experiences where we come close to feeling our 'spirit': highs, peak experiences, moments of deep peace, deep joy and connection, serendipity.'

In treating the 'whole person', herbalism acknowledges that stresses and imbalances in the body will have an effect on the mind and spirit, and vice versa.

Fortunately, Nature offers a vast medicine chest of remedies for all sorts of ailments, disorders and diseases, upon which we can all draw. Here follows a selection of recipes for various problems of the body, mind and spirit.

Most of these recipes use weights for dried herb amounts, because for medicines accuracy is particularly important. Many recipes also contain tinctures or mixtures of tinctures; these can be bought in, or made following the method in Key Preservation Techniques (pp.18–19).

With all of these recipes, consult your healthcare practitioner if symptoms persist or worsen. Conditions mentioned here may be transient or superficial, but in some cases they may be a sign of more serious illness, and lingering symptoms should always be investigated.

A note on doses

Adults

The recipes in this book all provide adult doses, as standard.

The standard dose of 5ml/1 tsp of tincture 3 times daily works well for chronic conditions; acute conditions (infections, for example) could warrant up to twice this amount over a shorter period.

See the advice on p.24 if you are pregnant, breastfeeding or have a serious or long-lasting health condition.

Children

As a general rule, children from ages 5 to 12 are given ¼ to ½ an adult dose. From ages 12 and up, they can be given an adult dose. That said, common sense should always prevail – some children are small for their age, some are big – and doses can be adjusted accordingly. It is good to use the minimal dose you need to get the desired effect.

Babies

Babies and young children aged 1–5 years should not be given tinctures. 1–5 tsps of tea or decoction can be given; ½ a tbs of syrups. At the time of writing this book, it was advisable not to give honey to babies under one year old.

Hot Stuff Circulation Stimulant

Feel warmer within minutes as these herbs zap round your bloodstream.

INGREDIENTS
Tinctures (pp.18–19):
- 10ml/2 tsp cayenne (p.156, Hot Cayenne Tincture)
- 10ml/2 tsp ginger
- 20ml/4 tsp prickly ash
- 20ml/4 tsp yarrow
- 20ml/4 tsp gingko
- 20ml/4 tsp hawthorn (p.75, Mother of the Heart Tincture)

MAKES & KEEPS
Makes a total of 100ml/just under ½ cup.
Keeps at least 3 years.

METHOD
Simply mix the tinctures together in a bottle.

Take ¼–½ tsp in warm water every 3–4 hours as it is needed.

Horse Chestnut & Broom Varicose Vein Lotion

This effective lotion is made in the form of a liniment (p.20) so it is easy to rub in over large areas.

INGREDIENTS
- 50ml/3 tbs + 1 tsp infused oil of broom tops (made with 2 tbs broom tops to 70ml/4 tbs + 2 tsp of olive oil, p.20)
- 50ml/3 tbs + 1 tsp tincture of horse chestnut seeds (conkers) (pp.18–19)

Essential oils:
- 20 drops rosemary
- 20 drops cypress

MAKES & KEEPS
Makes 100ml/just under ½ cup.
Keeps at least 1 year.

METHOD
Mix all the ingredients together in a bottle.

Shake before use. Apply twice daily, massaging a small amount into the legs from ankles upwards.

Vein-building Complex

Courtesy of Louise Idoux

Take internally to back up external treatment of varicose veins.

INGREDIENTS
Tinctures (pp.18–19):
- 30ml/2 tbs horse chestnut seeds (conkers)
- 25ml/5 tsp butcher's broom
- 10ml/2 tsp bilberry
- 10ml/2 tsp gingko
- 25ml/5 tsp buckwheat (made using leaves and flowers)

MAKES & KEEPS
Makes 100ml/just under ½ cup.
Keeps 2–3 years.

METHOD
Take ½–1 tsp 3 times daily in a little water.

Sinusitis & Infected Teeth Mix

Courtesy of Louise Idoux

A medicine to take internally to help fight infection.

INGREDIENTS
Tinctures (pp.18–19):
- 10ml/2 tsp fresh garlic
- 40ml/2 tbs + 2 tsp echinacea
- 10ml/2 tsp wild indigo
- 5ml/1 tsp goldenseal
- 15ml/1 tbs myrrh
- 20ml/4 tsp Pau d'arco

MAKES & KEEPS
Makes 100ml/just under ½ cup.
Keeps indefinitely.

METHOD
Mix the tinctures and bottle.

Take 1 tsp 3–5 times daily in a little water.

Heart & Blood Pressure Tea

Courtesy of Steve Kippax

Hawthorn helps to improve the efficiency of the heart as a muscle without increasing the oxygen used. Yarrow helps as a mild diuretic and by reducing blood pressure (you will need to take the tea for at least 6–8 weeks to experience this effect). Lime flowers are good as a relaxant, specifically affecting the heart.

INGREDIENTS
Equal parts of the following dried herbs:
- hawthorn flowering tops
- yarrow
- lime flowers

KEEPS
Keeps 1 year.

METHOD
Infuse 1 generous tsp of the dried herbs in a mug of water for 15 mins. Drink 3 times daily.

If one or other symptom is prevalent, then one or more of the herbs can be increased, up to double the original quantity.

— *Variation* —

IF YOU ADD AN EQUAL AMOUNT OF RED SAGE (DAN SHEN), THEN THE TEA MAY ALSO BE OF BENEFIT FOR CHEST PAIN/ANGINA-TYPE SYMPTOMS. IMPORTANT NOTE: IF YOU ARE TAKING WARFARIN OR OTHER PRESCRIPTION BLOOD-THINNING MEDICATIONS, YOU MUST CONSULT A HERBALIST, AS THIS FORM OF SAGE CAN POTENTIATE THE DRUGS AND THUS THE DOSAGE MAY NEED REVIEW. OTHER HERBS CAN ALSO BE OF BENEFIT FOR CARDIAC SYMPTOMS, BUT THEY ARE ONLY AVAILABLE FROM A QUALIFIED HERBALIST.

Bright Eyes Wash

This strong infusion is an effective eye wash for eye infections and sore eyes.

INGREDIENTS
Dried herbs:
- 15g/½oz marigold
- 15g/½oz eyebright
- 15g/½oz chickweed
- 15g/½oz roughly ground Oregon grape root
- 15g/½oz cornflowers

MAKES & KEEPS
Makes 75g/2½oz herb mixture, enough for 15 uses.
Keeps 1–2 years in dry form. Once made up, use the same day.

METHOD
Mix the herbs together.

Infuse 1 generous tbs in 250ml/1 cup boiling water. Leave to cool, then strain carefully through muslin or a thin cloth.

Wash the eyes 2–3 times daily using a sterile eye bath. Wash the eye bath well between each eye. Keep the eye wash covered between uses.

> **Caution**
> Always consult a healthcare professional for any eye problem.

Sage & Thyme Gargle

A simple, classic gargle mixture for sore throats and warding off colds.

INGREDIENTS
- 500ml/2 cups boiling water
- 25g/1oz sage leaves, dried or fresh
- 4 drops thyme essential oil

MAKES & KEEPS
Makes about 500ml/2 cups – enough for 10 gargles.
Keeps 3 days in the fridge.

METHOD
Pour boiling water on to the sage and leave until lukewarm. Strain and press through muslin or a thin cloth to get a very dark, strong infusion. Add the essential oil and bottle.

Shake well before use, then gargle with about 3 tbs. Repeat every hour in acute cases, otherwise use 3 times daily.

Coltsfoot Expectorant Honey

INGREDIENTS
- 1 large handful of coltsfoot flowers
- 500ml/2 cups water
- 320g/1 cup honey

MAKES & KEEPS
Makes 500ml/2 cups.
Keeps 1 year unopened. Once open, store in the fridge and use within 1 month.

METHOD
Decoct the flowers in water (p.15). Simmer uncovered to reduce to 250ml/1 cup of liquid. Strain and add an equal amount of honey.

Gently heat the mixture for a few minutes to dissolve the honey. Remove from the heat and pour into bottles.

Take 1 tsp 2–4 times daily for a cough.

Sinus-clearing Inhalation

INGREDIENTS
- 500ml/2 cups water, almost boiling
- 5ml/1 tsp benzoin tincture (Friar's Balsam)

Essential oils:
- 1 drop thyme
- 1 drop eucalyptus
- 1 drop lavender

MAKES & KEEPS
Makes 500ml/2 cups.
Use immediately.

METHOD
Put the ingredients into a large bowl. Carefully cover your head and the bowl with a towel so as to trap the steam inside. Inhale through the nose until there is no more steam.

Repeat every 4 hours as required.

— *Tip* —

FRIAR'S BALSAM TINCTURE LEAVES A RESIDUE OF RESIN ON THE SIDE OF THE CONTAINER THAT IS HARD TO WASH OFF. KEEP A CONTAINER ASIDE FOR FRIAR'S BALSAM USE ONLY, UNLESS YOU LIKE LOTS OF SCRUBBING!

Vapour Rub

Courtesy of Neil Williams

Rub into chest and neck to help relieve breathing and fight chest infections.

INGREDIENTS
- 90ml/just over $\frac{1}{3}$ cup + 2 tbs olive oil
- 1 tbs grated beeswax

Essential oils:
- 60 drops eucalyptus
- 60 drops pine
- 60 drops peppermint
- 60 drops cajeput
- 60 drops cedarwood

MAKES & KEEPS
Makes 100g/just under $\frac{1}{2}$ cup.
Keeps 1 year.

METHOD
Gently melt the beeswax into the olive oil in a double boiler or bain-marie. Let the mixture cool for 5 mins, then add the essential oils and pour into one or more jars.

Use sparingly.

> **Caution**
> Do not use on children under 2 years. Keep away from the eyes and delicate tissues.

Truly Tasty Cough Mixture

Courtesy of Geoff Edwards

INGREDIENTS

Dried herbs:
- 20g/¾oz coltsfoot
- 20g/¾oz Irish moss
- 20g/¾oz liquorice root
- 15g/½oz thyme
- 15g/½oz elecampane
- 15g/½oz white horehound

- 1.5 litres/1½ quarts water
- 35g/1¼oz ground marsh mallow root
- 1kg/36oz honey

Essential oils:
- 60 drops eucalyptus
- 60 drops aniseed
- 30 drops peppermint
- 2.5ml/½ tsp quillea fluid extract (p.18)

MAKES & KEEPS

Makes about 2 litres/2 quarts.
Keeps 1 year.

METHOD

Simmer all the dried herbs except for the marsh mallow root in the water for 30 mins, then strain. Measure the liquid and make up the volume to 1.25 litres/5¼ cups (add more water or reduce the liquid further, as required).

Meanwhile, make a smooth paste from the marsh mallow with a little water. Then add more water to make up to 500ml/2 cups.

Add to the herbal mix in the pan with the honey. Bring to the boil and bubble briskly for 5 mins. Remove from the heat and cool.

You should have about 2 litres/2 quarts of liquid. Separately, mix the essential oils and quillea tincture together (this emulsifies the essential oils so they do not separate), then add this to the rest.

Take 1–2 tsp 3–4 times daily, neat or with a little warm water.

Rosehip, Hawthorn & Pine Throat Lozenges

INGREDIENTS
- 3 generous handfuls of fresh rosehips
- 2 generous handfuls of fresh hawthorn berries
- up to around 500g/1½ cups golden syrup
- up to around 500g/2½ cups sugar
- 50ml/3 tbs + 1 tsp pine tincture (pp.18–19)
- 20 drops lemon essential oil

YOU WILL NEED
- SWEET MOULDS OR BAKING TRAY (P.22)

MAKES & KEEPS

Makes 100 or so sweets.
Keeps up to 6 weeks in a container in the fridge.

METHOD

Collect your berries, and immediately decoct in enough water to cover (p.15), covered, for 10 mins. Leave to cool. Mash up the mixture a little, then strain through a double layer of muslin. Mix this liquid (probably about 400ml/1⅔ cups) with equal amounts of both sugar and golden syrup.

Make into sweets (pp.21–22), stirring in the pine tincture and lemon essential oil just before pouring the mixture into moulds.

Lichen, Coltsfoot & Thyme Cough Sweets

INGREDIENTS
- 2 handfuls of lung lichen
- 500ml/2 cups water
- up to 400g/2 cups sugar
- up to 400g/1¼ cups golden syrup
- 50ml/3 tbs + 1 tsp coltsfoot tincture (pp.18–19)
- 20 drops thyme essential oil

YOU WILL NEED
- SWEET MOULDS

MAKES & KEEPS
Makes 100–200 small sweets.
Keeps up to 6 weeks.

METHOD
Make a decoction by bringing the lichen and water to the boil (p.15), then simmering for 10 mins with the lid on. Leave the mixture to cool, then strain.

Mix this liquid (about 400ml/1⅔ cups) with equal amounts of sugar and golden syrup. Make into sweets (pp.21–22), stirring in the coltsfoot tincture and thyme essential oil just before pouring the mixture into moulds.

Anti-nausea Tea

If you can keep it down, this can help with nausea.

INGREDIENTS
Dried herbs:
- 25g/1oz chamomile
- 25g/1oz peppermint
- 25g/1oz roughly ground root ginger

MAKES & KEEPS
Makes 75g/3oz herb mixture.
Keeps at least 1 year.

METHOD
Mix the herbs together and store in a jar.

Make the tea using 1 tsp per mug, infused for 5 mins.

Take 4–5 times daily.

Anti-nausea Suppositories

Courtesy of Dedj Leibbrandt

Use these when you feel too nauseous to take anything by mouth. The cocoa butter melts and releases the essential oils; these enter the blood stream and exert their medicinal effect.

INGREDIENTS
- 4 tsp cocoa butter

Essential oils:
- 12 drops chamomile
- 4 drops peppermint
- 4 drops lemon
- 1 drop ginger

YOU WILL NEED
- 7 x 2g suppository moulds

MAKES & KEEPS
Makes 7 suppositories.
Keeps 3 months in the fridge.

METHOD
Gently warm the cocoa butter in a double boiler or bain-marie until melted. Mix in the essential oils, pour into moulds and put in the fridge to set. Once set (usually after around 30 mins), remove from the moulds and store.

Insert 1 into your bottom as needed, or every 3–4 hours.

Marsh Mallow Water for Acid Indigestion

This is also good for coughs and catarrh.

INGREDIENTS
- 25g/1oz ground dried marsh mallow root (or 1 small handful of freshly dug roots)
- 500ml/2 cups cold water
- 1–2 tbs honey (optional; if using, manuka is the best)

MAKES & KEEPS
Makes 500ml/2 cups.
Keeps 3–4 days in the fridge.

METHOD
Soak the marsh mallow in the water for 30 mins. When softened, whizz up in a blender for a few minutes until smooth. Add the honey, if using, and leave to stand for 4 hours. Bottle and keep in the fridge.

Take 2 tbs 3 times daily until symptoms are finished.

THE RECIPES

Heartburn Tea

Courtesy of Steve Kippax

This tea is great for stomach pain, heartburn and reflux. The meadowsweet helps to reduce the inflammation in the stomach and marsh mallow root coats the stomach lining with a healing coat. Liquorice stops the pain and reflux associated with gastritis and heartburn.

INGREDIENTS
Dried herbs:
- 50g/2oz meadowsweet
- 50g/2oz marsh mallow root, ground
- 50g/2oz liquorice root, ground

MAKES & KEEPS
Makes 150g/6oz herb mixture.
Keeps 1–2 years.

METHOD
Mix the dried herbs together and store.

Take 1 generous tsp of the dried herbs infused in a mug of hot water for 15 mins 3–4 times daily.

Irritable Bowel Tincture Mix

Courtesy of Louise Idoux

INGREDIENTS
Tinctures (pp.18–19):
- 50ml/3 tbs + 1 tsp chamomile
- 10ml/2 tsp cardamom
- 15ml/1 tbs fennel
- 10ml/2 tsp wild yam
- 10ml/2 tsp cramp bark

MAKES & KEEPS
Makes 100ml/just under ½ cup.
Keeps 2–3 years.

METHOD
Simply mix and bottle.

Take 1 tsp in warm water 3 times daily.

Wind-reducing Syrup

For promoting good digestion and liver function.

INGREDIENTS
- 1 handful of fresh angelica root, roughly chopped (or 50g/2oz dried)
- 1 litre/1 quart water
- 340g/12oz jar of honey
- juice of 2 lemons

MAKES & KEEPS
Makes 640ml/22fl.oz.
Keeps up to 1 year in the fridge.

METHOD
Simmer the angelica for 2½ hours in the water. Strain and reduce to 300ml/1¼ cups of liquid. Add the honey and lemon juice. Gently warm and stir to dissolve the honey, then pour into bottles, tightening the lids when cool.

Take 1 tsp 1–3 times daily as required.

Anti-spasmodic Drops

Courtesy of Dedj Leibbrandt

A practitioner-level remedy for intestinal spasm consisting of a blend of tinctures. Measure using a millimetre measure — accuracy is important.

INGREDIENTS
Tinctures (pp.18–19):
- 10ml cramp bark (fluid extract if possible, p.18)
- 4ml pasqueflower
- 4ml yellow jasmine
- 2ml henbane

MAKES & KEEPS
Makes 20ml.
Keeps 2–3 years.

METHOD
Mix the tinctures together in a dropper bottle.

Take 10 drops in a little water every hour until spasms ease. Do not exceed 10 doses in 24 hours (see box below).

Always seek your healthcare practitioner's advice to determine the cause of pain.

> **Caution**
> Henbane and yellow jasmine are very strong herbs that are harmful in large doses. Very small amounts are used by herbal practitioners: a maximum of 5ml/1 tsp per week (equal to 5 drops taken 3 times daily). In the UK, only herbal practitioners are permitted to purchase these plants.

Worm Suppositories

Courtesy of Dedj Leibbrandt

For greatest success, use these alongside the Intestinal Parasite Treatment (p.104).

INGREDIENTS
- 4 tsp cocoa butter

Essential oils:
- 10 drops vetiver
- 10 drops oregano
- 5 drops cloves
- 5 drops roman chamomile

YOU WILL NEED
- 7 x 2G SUPPOSITORY MOULDS

MAKES & KEEPS
Makes 7 suppositories.
Keeps 3 months in the fridge.

METHOD
Gently melt the cocoa butter in a double boiler or bain-marie. Mix in the essential oils and pour into the moulds.

Insert 1 into your bottom evening and morning for 4 days either side of the new moon and full moon (when worms are most active).

Intestinal Parasite Treatment

Use these alongside the Worm Suppositories (p.103) for best effect.

INGREDIENTS
Tinctures (pp.18–19):
- 50ml/3 tbs + 1 tsp cloves
- 50ml/3 tbs + 1 tsp bayberry
- 50ml/3 tbs + 1 tsp wormwood
- 50ml/3 tbs + 1 tsp black walnut

To administer:
- 2 tsp linseeds/flax seeds
- 1 handful of pumpkin seeds (approx. 20)

MAKES & KEEPS
Makes 200ml/just over ¾ cup.
Keeps at least 2 years.

METHOD
Mix the tinctures together. Put 2 tsp of the tincture mix in 200ml/just over ¾ cup water.

To administer, grind the linseeds/flax seeds and mix them with the drink. Eat the pumpkin seeds, washing them down with the drink.

Do this once daily for 3 weeks. Leave for 1 week, then repeat for 2 weeks.

— *Tip* —

IF YOU CAN GET HOLD OF THEM, FRESH PAPAYAS CAN ALSO BE USED TO TREAT WORMS. TAKE 2 TSP FRESH PAPAYA SEEDS EVERY DAY FOR 3 WEEKS. CHEW THEM WELL.

Bowel Cleanse

Best used alongside a detox diet. If possible, eat a wholefood diet for at least 2–3 weeks before starting to take this mixture.

INGREDIENTS
Dried ground herbs:
- 50g/2oz yellow dock root
- 50g/2oz turkey rhubarb root
- 50g/2oz plantain leaves
- 50g/2oz Californian buckthorn bark
- 50g/2oz barberry bark

MAKES & KEEPS
Makes 250g/10oz (enough for 3 weeks).
Keeps 1 year.

Fresh:
- 2 tbs aloe vera gel
- 5cm/2in piece fresh root ginger, grated
- 4 garlic cloves, very finely chopped
- 1 litre/1 quart apple juice
- 2 tsp psyllium husks

MAKES & KEEPS
Makes 1 day's dose.
Use fresh.

METHOD
Thoroughly mix together the ground herbs.

Take 4 tsp of this mixture and add the aloe, ginger, garlic and apple juice. Mix well.

Take in the morning, adding the psyllium husks to the last ¼ of the liquid.

Drink daily for 3 weeks.

Do not give to children under 12 without professional advice.

Milk Thistle Liver Protector

Milk thistle has the ability to protect the liver from toxins, as well as to support a damaged liver while it regenerates.

INGREDIENTS
- 100g/4oz milk thistle seeds, dried and ground

MAKES & KEEPS
Makes 50–60 doses.
Keeps 1 year.

METHOD
Take 1 tsp stirred into ½ mug of warm water 1–2 times daily.

Bentonite Clay Cleanser

Clay is extremely absorbent, so it draws toxic substances. In the bowel, it will draw all kinds of toxins and help to eliminate them from the body.

INGREDIENTS
- 1 tsp clay
- 1 mug of chamomile tea (p.15)

MAKES & KEEPS
Makes 1 dose.
Drink immediately.

METHOD
Soak the clay in the chamomile tea for the day. Take on an empty stomach before bed.

Take daily for 3 weeks, then have a break for at least a week.

Coconut Liver Blast

This mixture is a good general boost for the liver, helpful alongside a detox diet. The mix is taken with coconut oil, which has been found to protect the liver from toxins.

INGREDIENTS
Dried ground herbs:
- 80g/3oz dandelion leaves
- 80g/3oz milk thistle seeds
- 80g/3oz angelica archangelica root
- 340g/12oz jar of virgin coconut oil

MAKES & KEEPS
Makes 580g/21oz.
Keeps at least 6 months.

METHOD
Gently melt the coconut oil in a double boiler or bain-marie and thoroughly mix in the herbs. Pour into a large jar and leave to set in a cool place for 30–60 minutes.

Take 1 tbs 1–2 times daily.

Cystitis Tea

INGREDIENTS

Dried herbs:
- 25g/1oz buchu leaves
- 25g/1oz plantain leaves
- 25g/1oz yarrow flowering tops
- 25g/1oz marsh mallow leaves

MAKES & KEEPS

Makes 100g/4oz herb mixture.
Keeps 1–2 years.

METHOD

Mix the herbs well. Make the tea, using 2 tbs to 1 litre/1 quart water (p.15).

Strain and drink over 1 day.

Repeat daily and continue for 5 days after the symptoms clear. Usually, the symptoms improve almost straight away, but if you stop taking the tea too soon, they will come back – the infection needs to be thoroughly cleared.

— *Tip* —

FOR CYSTITIS PREVENTION, TAKE 1 MUG OF CYSTITIS TEA, MADE FROM 1 TSP PER MUG, DAILY.

Cystitis Regime

Courtesy of Dedj Leibbrandt

INGREDIENTS

Tinctures (pp.18–19):
- 150ml/½ cup + 2 tbs cornsilk
- 75ml/¼ cup + 1 tbs buchu
- 75ml/¼ cup + 1 tbs bearberry

MAKES & KEEPS

Makes 300ml/about 1¼ cups.
Keeps 2–3 years.

METHOD

Put 100ml/just under ½ cup of the mixture into 1 litre/1 quart water.

Sip it over 24 hours and repeat the next day. On days 3 and 4, put 50ml/just under ¼ cup in 1 litre/1 quart water. Sip it over 24 hours. You must complete the 4-day course.

Do not give to children under 12.

> **Caution**
>
> If you don't feel better after the first 24 hours of this treatment, then you need antibiotics; see your doctor. Bladder infections must be treated quickly, as they can track up to the kidneys with serious consequences.

Waterfall Smoothie

Courtesy of Anne McIntyre

To help treat the retention of premenstrual fluid.

INGREDIENTS

75g/⅓ cup of the following fresh herbs:
- wild celery leaves
- dandelion leaves
- fennel leaves and/or seeds
- coriander leaves and/or seeds
- nasturtium leaves and flowers
- parsley leaves
- 1 bunch of celery, chopped
- 1 cucumber, chopped

YOU WILL NEED
- A BLENDER

MAKES & KEEPS
Makes 1 serving.
Drink immediately.

METHOD
Blend all the ingredients until smooth.

Drink the smoothie for breakfast first thing in the morning, and repeat throughout the day as often as desired. Continue over a few days, or over a few weeks if the problem is chronic.

Incontinence Tea

Helps to strengthen the bladder.

INGREDIENTS
Dried herbs:
- 25g/1oz horsetail
- 25g/1oz couchgrass
- 25g/1oz shepherd's purse
- 25g/1oz borage
- 25g/1oz marsh mallow leaves

MAKES & KEEPS
Makes 125g/5oz tea mix.
Keeps 1–2 years.

METHOD
Make the tea, using 2 tsp per mug (p.15).

Drink 2–3 cups daily.

Ladies' Lovelies

Courtesy of Sensory Solutions

These protective, nurturing and balancing drops help to support women of any age. They help with traumatic pregnancy and birth experiences and other female gynaecological issues, such as difficult menstruation, problems in conceiving and the menopause.

INGREDIENTS
- 30ml/2 tbs raspberry leaf tincture (pp.18–19)
- 30ml/2 tbs lady's mantle tincture (pp.18–19)
- 30ml/2 tbs nettle syrup (pp.21–22)

MAKES & KEEPS
Makes 90ml/just over ⅓ cup.
Keeps at least a year.

METHOD
Mix the ingredients together in a dropper bottle.

Take 5–10 drops 3–6 times daily as required.

Nettle Syrup

Delicious and rich in minerals and vitamin C.

INGREDIENTS
- 750ml/3 cups water
- 50g/2oz dried nettles (or 50g/2 cups fresh)
- 400g/2 cups sugar (I prefer brown or muscovado)

MAKES & KEEPS
Makes about 750ml/26fl.oz.
Keeps 3–12 months.

METHOD
Bring the water and nettles to the boil. Simmer for 10 mins with the lid on. Leave to steep for 3–4 hours, then strain.

Reduce the liquid to 500ml/2 cups. Add the sugar and boil for a further 4–5 mins, then pour into bottles.

Take 1–2 tsp daily as a mineral-rich syrup or use as a cordial.

PMS Chocolates

These bitter-sweet chocolates contain a daily dose of PMS-busting herbs.

INGREDIENTS
- 120g/½ cup cocoa butter
- 120g/½ cup coconut oil
- 120g/1 cup raw chocolate powder
- 2 tsp ground chasteberry (this herb tastes very bitter)
- 10g/⅓oz dried and ground lady's mantle
- approx. 2 tbs honey, agave syrup or maple syrup, to taste
- 1 handful of raspberries, dried or fresh
- 1 handful of chopped nuts
- 2 drops rose otto essential oil

YOU WILL NEED
- SMALL MOULDS, SUCH AS ICE-CUBE TRAYS

MAKES & KEEPS
Makes 40 ice-cube-sized chocolates.
Keeps 2–3 months in the freezer.

METHOD
Put all ingredients except the honey/syrup, raspberries, nuts and rose otto essential oil into a double boiler or bain-marie. Melt the butter over a very gentle heat, stirring constantly. Do not overheat. Add the honey/syrup to taste, and the raspberries and nuts, continuing to stir.

When you are satisfied with the sweetness, remove from the heat. Stir in the rose otto essential oil and pour it into the moulds. (Put about 1 tbs into each.)

Leave to set in the fridge for 30–60 minutes.

Eat 1 chocolate daily to help balance your hormones. You may use this remedy for 3–12 months. Don't stop and start; take continuously as the chasteberry works best that way.

When the PMS is most acute and you want to eat more chocolates, switch to No Stress Raw Chocolates (opposite).

No Stress Raw Chocolates

INGREDIENTS
- 120g/½ cup cocoa butter
- 120g/½ cup coconut oil
- 120g/1 cup raw chocolate powder
- 2 tbs ground valerian
- 4 tbs dried ground passion flower
- 2 tbs dried rose petals, broken into small pieces
- 1–2 tbs honey, agave syrup or maple syrup
- 2 drops rose otto essential oil
- 2 tbs cocoa nibs
- 2 tbs shelled hemp seeds

YOU WILL NEED
- SMALL MOULDS, SUCH AS ICE-CUBE TRAYS

MAKES & KEEPS
Makes 40 ice-cube-sized chocolates. Keeps 3 months in the freezer.

METHOD
Put all ingredients except the honey/syrup, rose otto essential oil, cocoa nibs and hemp seeds into a double boiler or bain-marie. Melt the cocoa butter over a very gentle heat, stirring constantly. Do not overheat. Add the honey/syrup to taste, continuing to stir.

When you are satisfied with the sweetness, remove from the heat. Stir in the rose otto essential oil, nibs and seeds, then pour it into the moulds. (Put about 1 tbs into each.)

Eat up to 4–5 daily in the days leading up to your period, or at any other stressful time.

Period Pain Chocolates

INGREDIENTS
- 120g/½ cup cocoa butter
- 120g/½ cup coconut oil
- 120g/1 cup raw chocolate powder
- 4 tsp ground cinnamon
- 4 tsp dried ground cramp bark
- 5 tsp skullcap
- 1–2 tbs honey, agave syrup or maple syrup
- 4 tbs cocoa nibs, shelled hemp seeds or chopped nuts

YOU WILL NEED
- SMALL MOULDS, SUCH AS ICE-CUBE TRAYS

MAKES & KEEPS
Makes 40 ice-cube-sized chocolates. Keeps 3 months in the freezer.

METHOD
Put all ingredients except the honey/syrup and nibs/seeds/nuts into a double boiler or bain-marie. Melt the cocoa butter over a very gentle heat, stirring constantly. Do not overheat. Add the honey/syrup to taste, continuing to stir.

When you are satisfied with the sweetness, remove from the heat, add the nibs/seeds/nuts and pour it into the moulds. (Put about 1 tbs into each.)

Eat 1 chocolate every 20 mins until period pain has eased, then 1 every 3 hours.

Period Pain Tea

Courtesy of Anne McIntyre

INGREDIENTS
Dried herbs:
- 50g/2oz rose
- 50g/2oz motherwort
- 50g/2oz lady's mantle
- 50g/2oz chamomile
- 50g/2oz clary sage

MAKES & KEEPS
Makes 250g/10oz herb mixture (enough for 10 days).
Keeps 1 year.

METHOD
Mix the herbs together. Place 50g/2oz of the herb mix in a teapot. Pour 1 litre/1 quart boiling water over the herbs and infuse for 10–15 mins.

Drink 1 mug 3 times daily throughout the month.

On the first day of the period, or whenever there is the most discomfort, drink throughout the day as needed, up to 6 mugs.

Cream for Vaginal Thrush

This versatile cream can also be used for men's thrush and for oral thrush.

INGREDIENTS
- 60g/¼ cup Heal-all Marigold Cream (p.81)

Essential oils:
- 6 drops tea tree
- 6 drops niaouli
- 6 drops palmarosa
- 2 drops oregano

MAKES & KEEPS
Makes 60g/¼ cup.
Keeps at least 6 months in the fridge.

METHOD
Mix the marigold cream and essential oils together.

Apply to the affected area 1–2 times daily.

Pessaries for Thrush

Courtesy of Dedj Leibbrandt

These help to soothe itching and restore vaginal health.

INGREDIENTS
- **32g/8 tsp cocoa butter**

Essential oils:
- **13 drops tea tree**
- **13 drops niaouli**
- **13 drops palmarosa**
- **4 drops oregano**

YOU WILL NEED
- 14 X 2G MOULDS

MAKES & KEEPS
Makes 14 pessaries.
Keeps 3 months in the fridge.

METHOD
Gently warm the cocoa butter in a double boiler or bain-marie until melted. Mix in the essential oils and pour into the moulds.

Insert 1 pessary as high as you can into the vagina 2 times daily. Lie down for 10–30 mins after inserting.

Morning Sickness Sweets

INGREDIENTS
- **½ handful of chopped fresh root ginger**
- **25g/1oz dried black horehound (double the quantity if fresh)**
- **450ml/just under 2 cups water**
- **550g/2¾ cups brown sugar**
- **60g/¼ cup butter (optional)**

YOU WILL NEED
- SWEET MOULDS

MAKES & KEEPS
Makes about 100 sweets.
Keeps 4–6 weeks in a container in the fridge.

METHOD
Boil the ginger and horehound in water for 20 mins. Strain and make the sweets (pp.21–22).

If using butter, add it just before pouring the sweet mix into the moulds.

Take 4–8 sweets daily, and enjoy.

FOR LABOUR

These are a few remedies to assist labour. All are tinctures unless otherwise stated, which can be bought in or homemade as instructed on pages 18–19. Always take tinctures by mixing them with water.

Please be aware that these remedies should only be used to assist birth where necessary, and should never be used in place of proper medical attention.

Labour Endurance Mix

To help keep one's strength up for labour.

INGREDIENTS
- 25g/1oz dried raspberry leaves
- 25g/1oz dried lady's mantle leaves
- 1 litre/1 quart boiling water
- 50ml/¼ cup Panax (American) ginseng tincture (pp.18–19)

MAKES & KEEPS
Makes 1 litre/1 quart.
Keeps 2 days.

METHOD
Make a tea from the raspberry leaves, lady's mantle leaves and water (p.15). Add the ginseng tincture. Sip throughout labour from the start.

Contractions Booster

To make weak contractions stronger, and to help expel the placenta.

INGREDIENTS
- golden seal tincture (pp.18–19) or dried ground root

METHOD
Take 1–2 tsp every 1–2 hours. If using the dried form, take ½–1 tsp. Note – it tastes vile!

Relaxing Mix for Labour

This is to take during labour if contractions are too strong and painful early on.

INGREDIENTS
Tinctures (pp.18–19):
- 15ml/1 tbs lobelia
- 40ml/2 tbs + 2 tsp blue cohosh
- 40ml/2 tbs + 2 tsp cramp bark
- 5ml/1 tsp yellow jasmine

MAKES & KEEPS
Makes 100ml/just under ½ cup.
Keeps 2–3 years.

METHOD
Take 1 tsp every 1–2 hours. If the cervix is not opening, take 1 tbs in a single dose.

Anti-haemorrhage Mix

This mixture can be used to slow any bleeding anywhere in the body.

INGREDIENTS
Tinctures (pp.18–19):
- 30ml/2 tbs yarrow
- 30ml/2 tbs shepherd's purse
- 30ml/2 tbs goldenseal

MAKES & KEEPS
Makes 90ml/6 tbs.
Keeps 2–3 years.

METHOD
Mix the tinctures together in a bottle.

Call an ambulance if medics are not already there. Take 4 tsp, followed by another 4 tsp in 15 mins if still bleeding.

No Sweat Sage Tea

Particularly useful for menopausal night sweats, sage can help any excessive sweating.

INGREDIENTS
- 3 tbs dried chopped sage leaves and flowers
- 1 litre/1 quart boiling water

MAKES & KEEPS
Makes 1 litre/1 quart (enough for 2 days). Keeps up to 3 days in the fridge.

METHOD
Place the sage in a teapot or lidded pan. Cover with the boiling water, add the lid and leave to cool. Strain and drink cold.

Take 1 mug 3 times daily for several weeks.

Syrupy Menopause Mix

A delicious way to take these female hormone-boosting herbs.

INGREDIENTS
- 120ml/½ cup wild yam root tincture (pp.18–19)
- 120ml/½ cup red clover syrup (pp.21–22)

MAKES & KEEPS
240ml/1 cup.
Keeps 1 year.

METHOD
Mix the tincture and syrup together and bottle. Take ½–2 tsp 2–3 times daily.

> **Note**
> Treatments for hormone conditions often take at least 3 months to take full effect.

Herbal 'HRT' Cream

This do-it-yourself cream is made from wild yam. Many women swear by it to help keep menopausal symptoms at bay.

INGREDIENTS
- 100ml/6 tbs + 2 tsp evening primrose oil
- 50g/½ cup emulsifying wax
- 200ml/¾ cup + 5 tsp wild yam root tea (p.15)
- 100ml/6 tbs + 2 tsp wild yam tincture (pp.18–19)

Essential oils (optional):
- 20 drops jasmine
- 20 drops neroli
- 20 drops clary sage
- 2ml/½ tsp benzoin tincture (Friar's Balsam)

MAKES & KEEPS
Makes approx. 450g/just under 2 cups. Keeps up to 1 year.

METHOD
Make as for Comfrey Cream for Speedy Healing (p.82), mixing in the essential oils, if using, with the benzoin.

To use, rub 1 tsp of the cream into soft skin (inside the arms, inner thighs, belly, breasts) 1–2 times daily.

Balancing Tincture for the Menopause

Courtesy of Anne McIntyre

INGREDIENTS

Dried herbs:
- 100g/4oz red sage leaves
- 100g/4oz motherwort
- 100g/4oz lady's mantle
- 100g/4oz chamomile
- 100g/4oz rose petals
  (or use 250g/9oz each of fresh herbs)
- 500ml/2 cups brandy or vodka

MAKES & KEEPS

Makes approx. 400ml/1⅔ cups tincture.
Keeps 2–3 years.

METHOD

Make a tincture from the ingredients (pp.18–19).

Take 1–2 tsp 3 times daily in a little water.

It may take 3 weeks–3 months to benefit fully.

Tea for Dizziness

INGREDIENTS

Dried ground herbs:
- 50g/2oz rosemary leaves
- 50g/2oz gingko leaves
- 50g/2oz wood betony leaves

MAKES & KEEPS

Makes 150g/6oz herb mixture.
Keeps 1–2 years.

METHOD

Mix well and store in a jar.

Make the tea as required, using 1 tsp per mug (p.15).

Take 3 mugs daily.

Cramp-relieving Tincture

Courtesy of Anthony Seifert

Helps to treat menstrual cramping and cramping due to dysentery, as well as headaches, sleeplessness and anxiety.

INGREDIENTS

Tinctures (pp.18–19):
- 45ml/3 tbs California poppy
- 30ml/2 tbs silk tassel
- 15ml/1 tbs lemon balm
- 15ml/1 tbs Jamaican dogwood bark

MAKES & KEEPS

Makes 105ml/just under ½ cup.
Keeps 2–3 years.

METHOD

Combine all the tinctures and bottle.

Take 10–30 drops up to 5 times daily until pain subsides.

Women's Balancing Tea (Swiss-style)

Courtesy of Christine Herren-Valette

This tea helps to harmonize the menstrual cycle.

INGREDIENTS

Dried ground herbs:
- 9g/3 tbs yarrow
- 6g/2 tbs raspberry leaf
- 6g/2 tbs lady's mantle
- 4g/2 tbs marigold flowers
- 5g/5 tsp sage

MAKES & KEEPS

Makes 30g/1oz herb mixture.
Keeps 1 year.

METHOD

Mix the herbs together. Make the tea (p.15), using 1 tsp of the herb mixture per mug of hot water.

Take 1–3 cups daily.

Herbal Tonic for Prostate Health

Many men suffer from prostate problems and can benefit from prostate-supporting herbs.

INGREDIENTS
Dried herbs:
- 15g/½oz nettle root
- 15g/½oz saw palmetto
- 15g/½oz horsetail
- 15g/½oz raspberry leaf
- 15g/½oz plantain
- 1 tbs white cedar

- 500ml/2 cups organic Apple Cider Vinegar (p.165) or organic vodka

MAKES & KEEPS
Makes approx. 400ml/1⅔ cups.
Keeps 2–3 years.

METHOD
Make a tincture or infused vinegar (pp.18–19).

Take 1 tsp 3 times daily in a little water.

— *Tip* —

TAKE 1–2 TBS PUMPKIN SEEDS DAILY TO BOOST YOUR ZINC LEVELS. PLENTY OF EXERCISE WILL ALSO HELP.

Men's Reproductive Tonic

May support in treating infertility and impotence.

INGREDIENTS
Dried ground herbs:
- 50g/2oz horsetail
- 50g/2oz damiana
- 50g/2oz ginseng

- 100g/¾ cup pumpkin seeds
- 340g/12oz jar of virgin coconut oil

MAKES & KEEPS
Makes 590g/22oz.
Keeps at least 1 year.

METHOD
Mix together the herbs and seeds. Separately, melt the coconut oil in a double boiler or bain-marie. Mix the herbs/seeds and oil together thoroughly and jar. Leave to set for 30–60 mins in a cool place. Once set, store in a cool place.

Take 1 tbs daily.

Anti-anxiety Drops with Valerian & Rose

INGREDIENTS
- 25g/1oz valerian root
- 12g/½oz rose buds
- 500ml/2 cups brandy
- 1 tbs honey

MAKES & KEEPS
Makes just under 500ml/2 cups.
Keeps 2–3 years.

METHOD
Mix all the ingredients together and put into a large jar with a lid. Leave in a cool place for 3 weeks. Strain and bottle.

Take 5–10 drops as required, up to 6 times daily.

Herbal Anti-depressant

This mix almost always lifts the spirits, without making you feel numb or interfering with painful emotions.

INGREDIENTS
Dried and powdered herbs:
- 75g/3oz oatstraw
- 75g/3oz rosemary
- 75g/3oz lemon balm
- 75g/3oz St John's wort
- 340g/12oz jar of runny honey or pure coconut oil

MAKES & KEEPS
Makes 640g/24oz.
Keeps 6–12 months.

METHOD
Mix the herbs together. Warm the honey or oil and mix well with the herbs. Pour into jars.

Take 1–2 tsp 1–3 times daily (if you feel very down, go for the higher dose of 2 tsp, then reduce it as you start to feel better).

False Solomon's Seal & Teasel for Joints

Courtesy of Matthew Wood

This acts on the carpals and tarsals and on the pelvic floor. It is also great for the small joints of the fingers if treating rheumatoid arthritis.

INGREDIENTS
Tinctures (pp.18–19):
- 60ml/¼ cup false Solomon's seal or 'dragon root'
- 60ml/¼ cup teasel

MAKES & KEEPS
Makes 120ml/½ cup.
Keeps 2–3 years.

METHOD
Mix the tinctures together in a bottle.

Take 3–5 drops 3 times daily.

Solomon's Seal & Agrimony Tension Remedy

Courtesy of Matthew Wood

This remedy for tension, both psychological and physical, relaxes most people in seconds. It's made with 7 parts agrimony to 4 parts Solomon's seal.

INGREDIENTS
Tinctures (pp.18–19):
- 210ml/¾ cup + 6 tsp agrimony (but make this with 1½ handfuls of fresh agrimony and 250–500ml/1–2 cups good brandy, enough to cover)
- 120ml/½ cup Solomon's seal (but make this with 1½ handfuls of Solomon's seal roots – unearthed, roughly chopped and placed in a jar – and 500ml/2 cups vodka)

MAKES & KEEPS
Makes approx. 500ml/2 cups.
Keeps at least 2 years.

METHOD
Mix the tinctures together in a bottle.

Take 3–5 drops 3 times daily (or as needed).

— *Tip* —

PICK THE AGRIMONY LEAVES OFF THE SIDES OF THE LEADER OR MAIN STEM, SO THAT THE LATTER CAN GO ON TO FLOWERING.

SOLOMON'S SALVES

The following variations on Solomon's seal salve come from the highly regarded US herbalist Matthew Wood. All feature the infused oil of true Solomon's seal root. To make this, use 200g/7oz dry plant material and enough safflower or olive oil to cover (around 250ml/1 cup) (p.20). To make each salve recipe, simply heat all the ingredients together until the beeswax has melted, stir and pour into jars.

All these recipes make 4 full 60ml/2oz jars, with possibly a little left over, and keep for at least 12 months in the fridge.

Apply these salves liberally to sore, affected areas 1–3 times daily.

Joint-aligning Salve

This helps to tighten loose joints and bring them back into alignment.

INGREDIENTS
- 200ml/¾ cup + 5 tsp infused oil of true Solomon's seal (see recipe above)
- 1600 IU vitamin E oil
- 40ml/2 tbs + 2 tsp Comfrey Oil (p.80)
- 3 tbs grated beeswax

Solomon's Bad Back Salve

This muscle and joint-relaxing salve has a particular affinity with the back.

INGREDIENTS
- 200ml/¾ cup + 5 tsp infused oil of true Solomon's seal (see recipe left)
- 1600 IU vitamin E oil
- 40ml/2 tbs + 2 tsp ginger root infused oil (p.20)
- 3 tbs grated beeswax

Salve for Dry Joints

Adding marsh mallow seems to enhance Solomon's seal's ability to moisten and nourish the joints.

INGREDIENTS
- 200ml/¾ cup + 5 tsp infused oil of true Solomon's seal (see recipe above left)
- 1600 IU vitamin E oil
- 40ml/2 tbs + 2 tsp marsh mallow root infused oil (p.20)
- 3 tbs grated beeswax

Cartilage-healing Salve

INGREDIENTS
- 200 ml/¾ cup + 1 tbs infused oil of true Solomon's seal (see recipe above left)
- 1600 IU vitamin E oil
- 40ml/2 tbs + 2 tsp horsetail tops infused oil (p.20)
- 3 tbs grated beeswax

Skin-calming Tea

This tea helps to soothe eczema and other itchy inflammations of the skin.

INGREDIENTS

Dried herbs:
- 25g/1oz red clover flowers
- 25g/1oz cleavers herb
- 25g/1oz ground dandelion root
- 25g/1oz dandelion leaf
- 25g/1oz nettle leaves
- 25g/1oz heartsease flowering tops
- 25g/1oz skullcap tops

MAKES & KEEPS
Makes 175g/7oz.
Keeps 1 year.

METHOD
Mix together equal parts of the above herbs. Store in a large jar.

Shake or mix well before each use. Make tea (p.15), using 2 tbs of the mixture infused in 3 mugs of boiling water for 7 mins.

Drink the 3 mugs over one day.

Take the tea for at least 3 months.

— *Tip* —

FOR ACNE, DRINK THIS TEA AND ALSO TAKE GARLIC AND ECHINACEA TINCTURE (PP.18–19), ½–1 TSP 3 TIMES DAILY. MOST PEOPLE WITH SKIN DISEASES ALSO NEED TO MAKE DIETARY CHANGES. DISCUSS THIS WITH YOUR HERBALIST OR HEALTHCARE PRACTITIONER.

Anti-fungal Ointment

Courtesy of Lynn Rawlinson

INGREDIENTS
- 100g/just under ½ cup coconut oil
- 60ml/¼ cup avocado oil

Essential oils:
- 8 drops lavender
- 8 drops neroli
- 4 drops myrrh
- 4 drops frankincense

MAKES & KEEPS
Makes 160g/⅔ cup.
Keeps 6–12 months.

METHOD
Gently melt the coconut oil with the avocado oil in a double boiler or bain-marie. Put the oil to one side to start to cool. When the oil starts to solidify, whisk and add the essential oils. Pour the mixture into glass jars.

Apply generously to the affected area twice daily until clear of infection.

Cold Sore Ointment

Courtesy of Lynn Rawlinson

INGREDIENTS
- 100g/just under ½ cup coconut oil
- 60ml/¼ cup avocado oil
- 5 drops lemon balm (melissa) essential oil

MAKES & KEEPS
Makes 160g/⅔ cup.
Keeps 6–12 months.

METHOD
Follow the method for Anti-fungal Ointment (above).

Apply a little to the affected area frequently.

Psoriasis Ointment

Courtesy of Lynn Rawlinson

Try a few different psoriasis treatments so that you find the best one for you.

INGREDIENTS
- 100g/just under ½ cup coconut oil
- 60ml/¼ cup avocado oil

Essential oils:
- 8 drops lavender
- 8 drops neroli
- 8 drops helichynum

- oil from 2 x 400 IU vitamin E capsules

MAKES & KEEPS
Makes 160g/⅔ cup.
Keeps 6–12 months.

METHOD
Follow the method for Anti-fungal Ointment (opposite). Then add both the essential oils and the vitamin E oil as the ointment cools.

Apply ointment generously to the affected areas 1–2 times daily.

— *Tip* —

PSORIASIS USUALLY NEEDS INTERNAL TREATMENT AS WELL. SEE THE SKIN-CALMING TEA OPPOSITE (TAKE THE TEA AS WELL AS USING AN EXTERNAL TREATMENT). A HERBALIST CAN USUALLY HELP PSORIASIS AND OTHER SKIN DISEASES WITH A TAILOR-MADE TREATMENT DESIGNED FOR YOU.

Psoriasis Cream

INGREDIENTS
- 120g/½ cup Heal-all Marigold Cream (p.81)

Essential oils:
- 7 drops neroli
- 7 drops lavender
- 7 drops bergamot

MAKES & KEEPS
Makes 120g/½ cup.
Keeps 6 months.

METHOD
Mix the essential oils into the cream.

Apply 2–3 times daily.

Psoriasis Lotion

If a large area of the body is affected by psoriasis, it is easiest to apply a lotion.

INGREDIENTS
- 100ml/just under ½ cup pure vegetable glycerine

Essential oils:
- 50 drops/½ tsp lavender
- 20 drops neroli
- 20 drops bergamot

- 100ml/just under ½ cup lavender water (bought in or homemade, p.15)

MAKES & KEEPS
Makes 200ml/just under ¾ cup.
Keeps up to 6 months.

METHOD
Whisk the essential oils into the glycerine, then gradually add the lavender water. Shake well before use.

Apply 2–3 times daily.

Acne Spot Ointment

Courtesy of Lynn Rawlinson

A variation on the Cold Sore Ointment (p.118).

INGREDIENTS
- 100g/just under ½ cup coconut oil
- 60ml/¼ cup avocado oil
- 8 drops tea tree essential oil

MAKES & KEEPS
Makes 160g/⅔ cup.
Keeps 6–12 months.

METHOD
Follow the method for Anti-fungal Ointment (p.118).

Apply frequently to spots.

Drawing Ointment

Courtesy of Neil Williams

Helps to draw out splinters or pus.

INGREDIENTS
- 25g/1oz dried marsh mallow root
- 90ml/just over ⅓ cup olive oil
- 25g/1oz dried slippery elm
- 1 tbs grated beeswax
- 30 drops lavender essential oil

MAKES & KEEPS
Makes 150g/just over ½ cup.
Keeps 1 year.

METHOD
In a double boiler mix the marsh mallow root in the olive oil. Simmer for 1 hour. Add the slippery elm and mix until smooth, then add the beeswax and allow to melt in. Let it cool slightly for 5 mins, and mix in the lavender oil before transferring to jars.

Apply generously to affected areas until the splinter or pus is out.

Fissure Salve

Courtesy of Stephen Buhner

Heals painful skin fissures (fingers, feet or anal) that do not respond to other interventions.

INGREDIENTS
- 28g/1oz Japanese knotweed root, dried and cut into tiny pieces
- 28g/1oz Stephania root (a Chinese vine with strong anti-inflammatory effects), dried and cut into tiny pieces
- 7g/¼oz dried thyme
- up to 500ml/2 cups olive oil, enough to cover
- ½ tsp vitamin E oil
- 3–6 tbs grated beeswax

MAKES & KEEPS
Makes up to 500ml/2 cups.
Keeps at least 1 year in the fridge.

METHOD
Make an infused oil (p.20) by putting the herbs in a lidded ovenproof dish and adding olive oil to cover to a depth of 1cm (½in). Leave overnight in the oven on its lowest setting.

Cool for an hour or so, strain and measure, then add the vitamin E oil and slowly reheat, adding 2 tbs of beeswax per 250ml/1 cup of oil.

Apply frequently.

KITCHEN PHARMACY

Cold Sore Lotion

Courtesy of Dedj Leibbrandt

INGREDIENTS

Tinctures (pp.18–19):
- 3ml/½ tsp myrrh tincture (this is made with 90%/190% alcohol because it is a resin; see tip, p.78).
- 4ml/¾ tsp lemon balm tincture
- 3ml/½ tsp St John's Wort Oil (p.83)
- 3 drops lemon balm (melissa) essential oil

MAKES & KEEPS
Makes 10ml/2 tsp.
Keeps 3 years.

METHOD
Mix together in a small bottle. Dab it on frequently throughout the day, reducing as the pain of the cold sore subsides.

Anti-wart Tincture

Courtesy of Karen Stephenson

INGREDIENTS
- 10g/⅓oz fresh greater celandine, crushed
- 250ml/1 cup Apple Cider Vinegar (p.165)

MAKES & KEEPS
Makes about 250ml/1 cup.
Keeps 1–2 years.

METHOD
Make as for herbal vinegars (p.19).

Dab undiluted on to warts twice daily. Alternatively, use a pad soaked in the tincture and place on to the wart with a bandage. Change daily.

Wart & Verucca Zapper

Courtesy of Dedj Leibbrandt

Suitable for adults and children, the zapper is good for clusters of warts or verrucas. Be aware that persistent warts or verrucas can indicate an underlying problem or weakness.

INGREDIENTS
- 5 tsp lemon essential oil
- 5 tsp castor oil
- 35ml/7 tsp white cedar tincture (pp.18–19)
- 15ml/3 tsp greater celandine tincture (pp.18–19)

MAKES & KEEPS
Makes 100ml/just under ½ cup.
Keeps 2–3 years.

METHOD
Mix all the ingredients together in a bottle.

Shake before each use. Cover the entire affected area twice daily. Note: it will take several weeks to take effect.

Fungal Toe Nail Cure

Courtesy of Dedj Leibbrandt

This treatment works if used for several months – and continued for 1 month after the nails look clear.

INGREDIENTS
Essential oils:
Mixture 1
- 50 drops/½ tsp cinnamon
- 1¼ tsp lemon
- 50 drops/½ tsp oregano

Mixture 2
- 1¼ tsp tea tree
- 50 drops/½ tsp thyme
- 50 drops/½ tsp palmarosa

MAKES & KEEPS
Makes 12ml/2½ tsp of each mixture.
Keeps 2–3 years.

METHOD
Rub mixture 1 into the nail bed once daily for 1 week. Then swap to mixture 2 and then back to mixture 1 and so on for as long as it takes to clear the nails.

Cancer Treatment Survival Drink

These herbs help the body to cope with the adverse effects of chemotherapy and radiotherapy.

INGREDIENTS
Dried ground herbs:
- 25g/1oz ginseng root
- 25g/1oz milk vetch root
- 25g/1oz ginger root
- 25g/1oz caraway seeds

MAKES & KEEPS
Makes 100g/4oz.
Keeps 1 year.

METHOD
Mix the ground herbs together and jar.

Make the tea (p.15), using 2 tsp per mug of boiling water. Infuse for 10 mins and drink 1 cup twice daily.

Alternatively, add 2 tsp of the herb mixture to your favourite smoothie.

Take it while having chemo and radiotherapy, and for a few months after to help the immune system recover.

Radiotherapy Healing Salve

Courtesy of Catherine Johnson

This is particularly good for women having radiotherapy for breast cancer. It maintains the skin's integrity and helps to prevent painful reddening of the skin.

INGREDIENTS
- 200ml/just over ¾ cup Heal-all Marigold Oil (p.81)
- 2¼ tbs grated beeswax
- 60 drops/½ tsp blue chamomile essential oil

MAKES & KEEPS
Makes 225g/just under 1 cup.
Keeps 6 months.

METHOD
Gently heat the marigold oil with the beeswax in a double boiler or bain-marie. Once melted, remove from heat, and allow to cool for 5 mins before stirring in the essential oil. Pour into a jar.

Gently apply to the skin over the affected area 3–4 times daily in the weeks prior to and during radiotherapy treatment.

> **Caution**
> Wash the skin before radiotherapy. Do not use salve for 2 hours before radiotherapy.

Blood-cleansing Formula

This mixture, for support during cancer treatment, is based on traditional cancer treatments (including the Native American 'Essiac' formula).

INGREDIENTS
Dried herbs:
- 100g/4oz burdock root, finely chopped
- 60g/2oz sheep sorrel leaves
- 20g/1¾oz slippery elm, ground
- 10g/⅓oz turkey rhubarb root

- 1 litre/1 quart boiling water
- 1 tbs ground turmeric

MAKES & KEEPS
Makes 190g/7¾oz herb mixture.
Keeps 1 year. Once made up, keeps 3 days in the fridge.

METHOD
Mix all the dry ingredients together, except the ground turmeric.

To make 1 day's dose, put 10g/⅓oz of the mixture with the water in a pan. Simmer, covered with a lid, for 10 mins. Remove from heat and leave overnight. The next day, bring back to the boil and add the turmeric powder. Leave off the heat for 15 mins, then strain.

Drink at least half straight away. Take the rest over the course of the day.

Violet Salve for Tumours

Courtesy of Louise Berliner

Violet leaves are known to dissolve hardness in the body. They are traditionally used to treat lumps in the breast.

INGREDIENTS
- 2 handfuls of fresh violet leaves (and flowers)
- 200ml/just over ¾ cup olive oil
- 5 tsp grated beeswax
- 1 drop of rose essential oil
- 10 drops frankincense essential oil

MAKES & KEEPS
Makes about 190g/¾ cup.
Keeps approx. 6 months.

METHOD
Pick the tiny violet leaves and flowers, and put them in a basket to wilt for a few hours. Make an infused oil over 5–6 weeks (p.20).

Strain off the oil and heat it gently with the beeswax in a double boiler or bain-marie to melt the wax. Then remove the mixture from the heat, add the rose and frankincense essential oils and pour into jars.

Apply a little to lumps 2–3 times daily.

> **Caution**
> Consult a healthcare professional right away if you find a lump in your breast, or elsewhere.

SNUFF

People have ingested herbs in ground form as a nasal snuff for millennia. It's a great strategy and can be a pleasant experience. The plant particles mop up infected reservoirs of mucus so that they can be expelled from the nose, while the good stuff in the herbs is absorbed straight into the blood stream. Snuffs are mostly used for problems with the nose and sinuses, but they also have some generalized effects on the body.

The method for making snuffs is always the same. Measure very finely ground herbs and mix together. Then rub in the essential oil (wear fine plastic gloves for hygiene). Sieve 8 times, using a very fine-mesh sieve, or more until the powders are blended and the essential oils mixed in.

Each recipe makes 6g/6 tsp of snuff and keeps at its best for 1 year. Store in a small airtight container. Take a pinch of snuff and sniff it up the nose 2–3 times daily.

All these recipes are courtesy of Melissa Ronaldson.

Uplifting Snuff

To uplift the mood.

INGREDIENTS
- 2g/2 tsp marsh mallow root
- 2g/2 tsp rosemary
- 2g/2 tsp sweet flag
- 1 drop frankincense essential oil

Soothing Snuff

Calms sore and inflamed sinuses.

INGREDIENTS
- 2g/2 tsp marsh mallow root
- 2g/2 tsp plantain
- 2g/2 tsp echinacea
- 1 drop chamomile essential oil

Opening & Clearing Snuff

Helps to open sinuses and clear blocked mucus.

INGREDIENTS
- 2g/2 tsp marsh mallow root
- 2g/2 tsp lime flowers
- 2g/2 tsp elecampane

Essential oils:
- 1 drop peppermint
- 1 drop eucalyptus

Polyp Snuff

To shrink nasal polyps.

INGREDIENTS
- 2g/2 tsp marsh mallow root
- 2g/2 tsp myrica
- 2g/2 tsp oak bark
- 1 drop frankincense essential oil

Up-all-night-&-still-dancing Snuff

These herbal stimulants help to keep you going longer.

INGREDIENTS
- 2g/2 tsp marsh mallow root
- 2g/2 tsp ashwaganda
- tiny pinch of black pepper
- tiny pinch of chilli pepper
- 2 drops peppermint essential oil

BABIES' & CHILDREN'S RECIPES

Here follow some safe and effective recipes for treating children and babies. All of these recipes are also suitable for adults; an adult dose is up to double the children's one.

Some of these recipes contain honey, but please note it's not recommended that you give honey to babies under 1 year old. Always consult your healthcare practitioner for any serious symptoms in young people.

Dry-bed Syrup

INGREDIENTS
- 15g/½oz dried agrimony (or 30g/1oz fresh)
- 15g/½oz dried St John's wort (or 30g/1oz fresh)
- 30g/1oz fennel seeds
- 500ml/2 cups water
- 240g/12oz jar of honey

MAKES & KEEPS
Makes approx. 700ml/24fl.oz.
Keeps 1 year unopened. After opening, keep in fridge and use within 1 month.

METHOD
Decoct the herbs in the water (p.15). Simmer the decoction for 10 mins, then leave to steep until cool. Strain. Add the honey and return to the heat to make a syrup (pp.21–22).

Give 1 tsp at bedtime until the bed-wetting problem is resolved.

Wild Cherry Cough-calming Syrup

INGREDIENTS
- 50g/1 cup wild cherry root
- 500ml/2 cups water
- 250ml/1 cup cherry juice (freshly made or bought in)
- 400g/2 cups white sugar

MAKES & KEEPS
Makes approx. 800ml/27fl.oz.
Keeps 1 year unopened. After opening, keep in fridge and use within 1 month.

METHOD
Decoct the wild cherry root in the water (p.15). Simmer the decoction until reduced by about half (this usually takes around 20–30 mins). Strain and add the cherry juice and sugar. Make the syrup (pp.21–22).

Give ½–2 tsp at night to help sleep. Also give ½–1 tsp up to 3 times a day to calm an irritable cough (when no mucus needs to be coughed up; see box below).

> **Caution**
> The syrup suppresses coughing, which is helpful at night. However, if there is mucus that needs to be coughed up from the lungs, do not use this mixture during the day, as coughing then will rid the lungs of mucus.

Children's Cough Honey

Courtesy of Anne McIntyre

INGREDIENTS
- 340g/12oz jar of runny honey
- 4g/2 tsp holy basil leaves
- 4g/2 tsp thyme leaves
- 4g/2 tsp hyssop flowering tops

MAKES & KEEPS
Makes approx. 340g/12oz.
Keeps at least 1 year.

METHOD
Remove some of the honey so that the jar is ⅘ full. Place the herbs in a reusable tea bag (or tie them in a small piece of muslin) and add to the jar. Leave on a sunny windowsill for 3 weeks. If you want a stronger flavour, remove the bag and replace it with the same quantity of fresh herbs, then infuse for another few weeks.

Give 1 tsp daily in a mug of hot water or ginger tea (p.15) as a preventative. Give 3–6 times daily in acute infections.

Cough Tea

This is a good alternative to cough honey (above), which is suitable for babies under 1 year of age.

INGREDIENTS
Dried herbs:
- 25g/1oz holy basil leaves
- 25g/1oz thyme leaves
- 25g/1oz hyssop flowering tops

MAKES & KEEPS
Makes 75g/3oz herb mixture.
Keeps 1 year.

METHOD
Mix the herbs together and store in a jar.

Make the tea (p.15), using 1 tsp herb mix to 1 mug of boiling water. Place the herbs in a teapot and add boiling water. Infuse for 10 mins.

Drink while warm, 1–3 cups daily.

Baby's First Herbal Tea

This tea both soothes and calms the digestive system and gets baby used to herbal teas.

INGREDIENTS
One or more of the following dried herbs:
- 25g/1oz chamomile flowers
- 25g/1oz fennel seeds
- 25g/1oz lime flowers

MAKES & KEEPS
Makes 1 serving.
Keeps 1 year.

METHOD
Make a weak infusion (p.15), using 1 tsp per mug of boiling water, brewed for 5 mins and then strained.

Leave to cool and give 1–2 tsp to baby on a teaspoon. (You can drink the rest.)

Any baby who can sip from a teaspoon is old enough for this tea. It can be served every day.

Salve for Eczema

Courtesy of Anne McIntyre

INGREDIENTS
- 300ml/1¼ cups coconut oil
- 1 handful of a mixture of marigold petals, chamomile flowers and lavender flowers (ideally fresh), roughly chopped

MAKES & KEEPS
Makes 300ml/1¼ cups.
Keeps 3–6 months.

METHOD
Gently heat the oil and the herbs in a double boiler or bain-marie for 3–4 hours. Strain and press through muslin. Discard the herbs and pour the liquid into jars.

Apply generously to the affected area at night and morning, after gently washing the area with rosewater.

Meadowsweet Anti-diarrhoea Honey

Raw honey's antibacterial properties can help to treat diarrhoea. Combined with astringent, anti-inflammatory meadowsweet, it makes a delicious and useful remedy for infants' and children's diarrhoea.

INGREDIENTS
- 340g/12oz jar of honey
- an equal amount of strong meadowsweet tea (p.15; make with 360ml/1½ cups boiling water over 25g/1oz dried meadowsweet/1 handful of fresh)

MAKES & KEEPS
Makes 680g/24oz.
Keeps up to 1 year unopened. Once opened, keep in the fridge and use within 1–2 months.

METHOD
Add the honey to the hot tea, stirring well until it all has dissolved. Bottle.

Give 1 tsp every 1–2 hours to treat an attack of diarrhoea. Continue to give 2 tsp daily for 5 days after the attack has passed.

> **Caution**
> Children can very quickly become dehydrated if they have diarrhoea. Replenish lost fluids with the 'Lemon Sherbert' Rehydration Remedy (p.93) and seek healthcare advice.

Mucus-busting Tea

Courtesy of Anne McIntyre

INGREDIENTS
Dried herbs:
- ½ tsp chamomile flowers
- ½ tsp plantain leaves
- ½ tsp elderflowers
- 500ml/2 cups boiling water

MAKES & KEEPS
Makes approx. 400ml/1¾ cups.
Keeps 4 days in the fridge.

METHOD
Mix the herbs together. Pour on the boiling water and leave to cool. Strain.

Give 2 tbs in a bottle or 6 tsp off a spoon before feeding, 3 times daily.

Teething Rub

Courtesy of Anne McIntyre

INGREDIENTS
- 1 tsp dried chamomile flowers
- 1 mug of boiling water

MAKES & KEEPS
Makes 1 mug.
Keeps 4 days in the fridge.

METHOD
Infuse the flowers in the water (p.15) for 1 hour until cool.

Strain and soak a teething ring or cloth in the cold tea.

Give to the baby to suck, or rub on to sore gums, as needed.

Sore Throat Gargle

Courtesy of Anne McIntyre

Many children love to gargle once they are old enough – which could be as young as 4 or 5, depending on the child.

INGREDIENTS
- ½ tsp ground turmeric
- ½ tsp sea salt
- 1 mug of warm water

MAKES & KEEPS
Makes 1 mug, enough for 1 day.
Keeps up to 3 days in the fridge.

METHOD
Dissolve the turmeric and salt in the water.

Gargle frequently throughout the day.

Sweet Sleep Syrup

Helps a fractious child relax into sleep.

INGREDIENTS
Dried herbs:
- 25g/1oz chamomile
- 15g/½oz catnip
- 15g/½oz rose buds or petals

- 500ml/2 cups rosewater
- 400g/2 cups sugar, or 1¼ cups honey

MAKES & KEEPS
Makes approx. 600ml/20fl.oz.
Keeps 6–12 months in the fridge.

METHOD
Mix all the herbs together in a pan and add the rosewater. Bring the mixture to the boil, then remove from the heat. Leave to cool, then strain. Reduce the liquid to 300ml/1¼ cups by simmering. Make a syrup with the sugar or honey (pp.21–22).

Give 1–3 tsp in a mug of hot milk or almond milk at bedtime.

Sweet Sleep Pillow for Children

INGREDIENTS
Dried herbs:
- 40g/1½oz lime flowers, finely shredded
- 20g/¾oz lavender flowers
- 20g/¾oz rose petals

Essential oils:
- 5 drops lavender
- 3 drops rose

YOU WILL NEED
- APPROX. 30CM X 20CM/12IN X 8IN RECTANGULAR BAG OF COTTON CLOTH/SMALL PILLOW CASE

MAKES & KEEPS
Makes 1 pillow.
Keeps effective for 6 months or more.

METHOD
Mix the herbs well in a large bowl. Sprinkle on the oils. To make the pillow, fill the bag/pillow case with the mix and ensure it's sealed.

Place the herbal pillow beside the child's ordinary pillow.

— *Tip* —

REFRESH THE PILLOW BY ADDING A FEW DROPS OF ESSENTIAL OILS EVERY NOW AND THEN, TO KEEP IT SMELLING LOVELY. AS AN ALTERNATIVE TO A PILLOW, MAKE A 'TRANQUIL TEDDY' BY STUFFING A FAVOURITE CUDDLY TOY WITH EITHER OF THE SLEEP PILLOW HERB MIXTURES (ABOVE AND OPPOSITE). REPLACE THE HERBAL MIXTURE AFTER 6–12 MONTHS.

Holy Sleep Pillow

Courtesy of Anne McIntyre

Promotes sleep and pleasant dreams.

INGREDIENTS
Dried herbs:
- 25g/1oz lavender flowers
- 50g/2oz chamomile flowers
- 25g/1oz holy basil

YOU WILL NEED
- ABOUT 12 X 8-INCH RECTANGULAR BAG OF COTTON CLOTH/SMALL PILLOWCASE

MAKES & KEEPS
Makes 1 pillow.
Keeps effective for 6 months or more.

METHOD
Make and use as for the Sweet Sleep Pillow for Children (opposite).

— *Tip* —

YOU COULD ALSO PLACE THE HERBS LOOSE IN A BOWL BY YOUR BEDSIDE.

Calming Herbal Baths

Courtesy of Anne McIntyre

This bath can be used daily or when a child is fussy, in pain or discomfort — or simply over-energized.

INGREDIENTS
Use 1 generous handful of any of these herbs (or mix any two or more of them):
- chamomile flowers
- lavender buds
- rose petals
- lemon balm leaves

YOU WILL NEED
- A STOCKING OR THIN SOCK

MAKES & KEEPS
Makes enough for 1 bath. If using dried herbs, you can prepare in advance; the dry mix will keep for 1 year.

METHOD
Place the herbs in a stocking or thin sock and knot it at the end to make a herbal bath bag. Tie it so that the hot water runs over it as you fill the bath. Fill the bath completely with hot water, then let it cool to a comfortable temperature. Squeeze the herbal bath bag to increase the strength of the infusion.

Sesame & Lavender Baby Oil

Courtesy of Anne McIntyre

INGREDIENTS
- 120ml/½ cup sesame oil
- 30 drops lavender essential oil

MAKES & KEEPS
Makes 120ml/½ cup.
Keeps 6–12 months.

METHOD
Mix the ingredients together.

Apply gently over the baby's skin. Avoid contact with the eyes.

Soothing Oat Bath

A soothing alternative to bubble bath, good for any kind of itching or irritated skin. It also soothes chickenpox sores.

INGREDIENTS
- 100g/1 cup oatmeal or porridge oats

YOU WILL NEED
- A SOCK

MAKES & KEEPS
Makes 1 bath.
Keeps dry for 3–6 months in the bathroom.

METHOD
Place the oats in the sock. Tie it round the hot tap so that the water runs through the oats as it fills the bath. Allow the water to cool to a comfortable temperature.

— Variation —

FOR A CALM AND SOOTHING BATH, ADD SOME OF THE HERBS SUGGESTED FOR THE CALMING HERBAL BATHS (P.129) TO THE OATS.

Rash Ointment

Courtesy of Teri Evans

This will nourish your hands as well as your baby's bottom.

INGREDIENTS
Dried herbs:
- 1 tbs chickweed leaves
- 1 tbs marsh mallow root
- 1 tbs comfrey root or leaf
- ½ tsp golden seal or baical skullcap flowering tops
- 225ml/just under 1 cup sweet almond oil
- 6 tbs grated beeswax

MAKES & KEEPS
Makes 220ml/just under 1 cup. Keeps 2 months.

METHOD
Infuse the herbs with the almond oil (p.20). Gently cook for 2–3 hours in a double boiler. Strain, melt in the beeswax and pour into jars.

Apply every time you change a nappy.

Vitamin Ice Lollies

A good way to get healthy herbs into your child.

INGREDIENTS
- 75ml/⅓ cup Many Berry Cordial (p.55)
- 350ml/1½ cups cooled nettle tea (p.15; make with 4 tsp nettles infused in 400ml/1⅔ cups boiling water for 10 mins)

YOU WILL NEED
- ICE-LOLLY MOULDS

MAKES & KEEPS
Makes 8–10 lollies. Eat within 3 months.

METHOD
Mix the ingredients together. Pour into ice-lolly moulds and freeze.

Eat 1–2 daily.

Anti-allergy Ice Pops

These can help to treat hayfever and pet allergies.

INGREDIENTS
- 350ml/1½ cups nettle leaf tea (make as for Vitamin Ice Lollies, opposite)
- 75ml/⅓ cup elderflower syrup (pp.21–22)

YOU WILL NEED
- ICE-LOLLY MOULDS OR ICE-CUBE TRAYS

MAKES & KEEPS
Makes 16–20 ice pops.
Eat within 3 months.

METHOD
Mix the ingredients well. Freeze in ice-lolly moulds or ice-cube trays.

Eat 1–3 daily.

Special Baby Wipes

Courtesy of Anna Dowding

These guarantee a permanently peachy bottom …

INGREDIENTS
- 2 tsp best-quality Apple Cider Vinegar (p.165)
- 2 tsp calendula tincture (pp.18–19)

Essential oils:
- 3–4 drops tea tree
- 3–4 drops lavender
- 2 tsp vegetable oil (either coconut, jojoba or olive)
- 500ml/2 cups of water

YOU WILL NEED
- COTTON WIPES OR COTTON WOOL

MAKES & KEEPS
Makes 100–200 wipes. Keeps 6 months or more.

METHOD
Mix all the ingredients together in a litre/quart jar. Squash in as many wipes or cotton wool balls as you can to soak up the mixture. Close the jar and keep it sealed until use.

Baby Powder for a Dry Bottom

A herbal alternative to talcum powder.

INGREDIENTS
- 4 tsp cornflour
- 3 tbs bicarbonate of soda
- 2 tbs dried chamomile flowers, ground to a fine powder
- 5 drops lavender essential oil

MAKES & KEEPS
Makes 90g/just over ½ cup.
Keeps up to 6 months in an airtight container.

METHOD
Mix all the ingredients together. Sift the mixture a couple of times. Shake well before use.

— Variation —

FOR A STRONG POWDER TO HELP PREVENT AND TREAT ATHLETE'S FOOT, ADD ESSENTIAL OILS (30 DROPS TEA TREE AND 30 DROPS LAVENDER) TO THE MIXTURE.

Antioxidant-rich Sunscreen

Courtesy of Monika Ghent

This makes a moderately strong sunscreen.

Read the section on cream-making techniques (pp.20–21) before you start.

INGREDIENTS
Oil phase:
- 40ml/2 tbs + 2 tsp olive oil
- 60g/¼ cup coconut oil
- 20g/4 tsp shea butter
- 7.5ml/1½ tsp liquid lecithin
- 1½ tsp grated beeswax

Water phase:
- 15ml/1 tbs fresh aloe gel
- 60ml/¼ cup green tea infusion (p.15)
- 45ml/3 tbs rosewater
- 20 drops carrot seed oil

Essential oils:
- 30 drops lavender essential oil
- 5 drops rosemary
- 5 drops peppermint

- 10 drops liquid vitamin D
- 5 x 400 IU vitamin E capsules
- 10 drops Walnut Flower Remedy (p.59)
- 10g/3 tsp zinc oxide

YOU WILL NEED
- A HAND BLENDER

MAKES & KEEPS
Makes 260g/1 cup.
Keeps 1–3 months in the fridge.
Refrigerate between uses.

METHOD
Measure all the ingredients and have them ready to use before you begin.

Melt the oil phase ingredients in a double boiler. Put the aloe gel into a bowl and whip it into a foam with a hand blender. Slowly drizzle the oil phase into the water phase. Blend well together for a couple of minutes.

Add the carrot seed oil, essential oils, vitamin D, vitamin E, Walnut Flower Remedy and zinc oxide to the cream while blending.

Nit Treatment for Kids

Use this together with a good nit comb.

INGREDIENTS
- 250ml/1 cup strong double decoction of quassia bark (p.15)
- 50 drops/½ tsp tea tree essential oil (not suitable for children under 7 years)

MAKES & KEEPS
Makes about 250ml/1 cup.
Enough for a 3-day treatment.
Use immediately.
Keeps up to 4 days in the fridge.

METHOD
Mix the ingredients together, only adding the tea tree essential oil if treating anyone over 7 years.

Wash the hair and apply lots of conditioner, then comb through with a nit comb.

Rinse hair, towel dry and apply the treatment all over the head from root to tip. Wrap up in a towel and leave to dry.

Repeat daily for 3 days, and then again after 5 days. Note: everyone in the house needs to be treated.

— *Tip* —

YOU MIGHT LIKE TO USE 125 ML/ ½ CUP OF THIS DECOCTION TO MAKE THE NIT-DETERRING CONDITIONER (P.206).

AROMATIC WATERS

Distilling aromatic waters is great fun – your kitchen will soon resemble an inventor's laboratory! You can either purchase a small copper still, or make your own. Aromatic waters are wonderful products to use in foods, to take as medicines and aids for well-being and to use on the skin, whether alone or as part of other recipes. If taken as medicines, the adult dose for aromatic waters is 2 tsp 3 times daily.

All these recipes are courtesy of Joe Nasr.

Peppermint Water

This delicious aromatic water is perfect for treating heartburn and indigestion, and as a cooling lotion if applied to the skin.

INGREDIENTS
- 150g/5oz dried peppermint (or 300g/10oz fresh)
- 2.5 litres/2½ quarts water

MAKES & KEEPS
Makes 300ml/1¼ cups.
Keeps at least a year.

METHOD
Place the peppermint and the water together in the pressure cooker. Make following the instructions for Gripe Water (right).

Gripe Water

Primarily to give to babies for colic, but anyone with indigestion can take this.

INGREDIENTS
Dried herbs:
- 60g/2oz aniseed
- 60g/2oz fennel seeds
- 30g/1oz dill seeds
- 2.5 litres/2½ quarts water

YOU WILL NEED
- PRESSURE COOKER
- 5MM/¼IN SILICONE HOSE (FROM BREWER'S HARDWARE)
- POSSIBLY A HOT PLATE, DEPENDING ON THE POSITION OF YOUR COOKER

MAKES & KEEPS
Makes 300ml/1¼ cups.
Keeps at least a year.

METHOD
Place the seeds and water in a pressure cooker on a worktop near the sink (use a hotplate if necessary). Close the lid and remove the pressure regulator to expose the vent pipe (steam exit).

Connect the hose to the vent pipe. Pass the hose beneath the water tap and then on and into a collecting glass bottle (300ml/10fl.oz).

Turn on the heat to high. When the water boils, open the tap to allow cold water to flow around and cool the hose.

Simmer on a low heat. To obtain a good-quality water, the distillation process should be slow with minimum heat; the distillate should not be warm to the touch but cool, ideally 35°C/95°F. Simmer until you have distilled 300ml/1¼ cups of gripe water (which in a household pressure cooker should take around 30–45 mins).

Infants: Give 10–20 drops in water or milk up to twice daily.

Breast-feeding mothers: Take 1–1½ tsp 3 times daily after meals.

Adults: Take 1–2 tsp for indigestion.

Lavender Water

Aromatic water of lavender can be used on its own as a healing and calming tonic (for inside and outside the body), or added to other recipes.

INGREDIENTS
- 150g/5oz dried lavender flowers (300g/10oz of fresh)
- 2.5 litres/2½ quarts water

MAKES & KEEPS
Makes 300ml/1¼ cups.
Keeps at least 1 year.

METHOD
Make in the same way as for Gripe Water (p.133).

— *Variation* —

YOU COULD SUBSTITUTE HALF THE LAVENDER FOR ROSE BUDS TO MAKE ROSE AND LAVENDER WATER.

Rosemary Water

A delicious flavouring for foods, this is also a hair tonic, a toner for the skin and a medicine to help circulation and memory.

INGREDIENTS
- 150g/5oz dried rosemary (300g/10oz of fresh)
- 2.5 litres/2½ quarts water

MAKES & KEEPS
Makes 300ml/1¼ cups.
Keeps 2 years.

METHOD
Make as for Gripe Water (p.133).

Lemon Balm Water

This lovely, lemony water uplifts the mood, helps treat headaches and is an anti-viral. It is especially good against the herpes viruses.

INGREDIENTS
- 150g/5oz dried lemon balm (300g/10oz of fresh)
- 2.5 litres/2½ quarts water

MAKES & KEEPS
Makes 300ml/1¼ cups.
Keeps 6 months.

METHOD
Make as for Gripe Water (p.133).

Rose & Chamomile Water

This is a soothing skin lotion, great as a spray for urticaria and for sore skin, including sunburn. It can be taken internally for the stomach and the womb.

INGREDIENTS
- 100g/4oz dried chamomile flowers
- 100g/4oz dried aromatic rose (must be organic)
- 2.5 litres/2½ quarts water

MAKES & KEEPS
Makes 300ml/1¼ cups.
Keeps for 6 months.

METHOD
Make as for Gripe Water (p.133)

PETS' CORNER

Animals can be treated similarly to people, although some animals should not have some herbs. Only use these recipes for the specified animals, unless advised otherwise by a specialist vet. These recipes are safe for home use; if in doubt, always consult a qualified holistic vet.

For the tinctures provided by holistic vet Barbara Jones, either buy in the tinctures, or make your own according to the method given in the Key Preservation Techniques, pages 18–19. They all keep for 2 years or more. For all the tinctures, mix together in a bottle and use as instructed.

Valerian & Catnip Cat Toy

Cats love the smell of these herbs, particularly the valerian.

INGREDIENTS
- 1 tbs dried valerian root, finely chopped
- 1 tbs catnip

YOU WILL NEED
- MATERIAL AND A SEWING KIT TO MAKE A SMALL TOY 'MOUSE'

MAKES & KEEPS
Makes 1.
Your cat will hunt the mouse down before it goes off!

METHOD
Mix the herbs well. Sew a mouse-shaped small bag, leaving the tail end open. Stuff it full with the herb mixture.

Sew up tightly and add a string 'tail' to the mouse.

Mange Treatment for Animals

Courtesy of Dedj Leibbrandt

This stinks, but works!

INGREDIENTS
- 3 heads garlic, roughly chopped
- 2 handfuls of fresh elder leaves and stems, finely chopped
- 2 litres/2 quarts water

MAKES & KEEPS
Makes about 1.5 litres/1½ quarts.
Keeps 4–5 days in the fridge.

METHOD
Simmer the herbs in the water for 10 minutes. Remove from the heat and leave overnight. Then strain and bottle.

Apply directly to affected areas twice daily until free of mange.

Animal Eardrops

Courtesy of Barbara Jones

INGREDIENTS
- 40ml/2 tbs + 2 tsp mullein oil (p.20)
- 2 drops thyme essential oil
- 1 tsp Heal-all Marigold Oil (p.81)
- 1 tsp garlic infused oil (p.20; make by infusing 2 crushed garlic cloves in 2 tsp vegetable oil, leave for 1–2 weeks, then strain)

MAKES & KEEPS
Makes 50ml/just under ¼ cup.
Keeps 6 months.

METHOD
Mix the ingredients together in a dropper bottle for easy use.

Put 2 drops into the animal's ears twice a day.

Scratch Pet Flea Remedy for Cats & Dogs

Courtesy of Louise Idoux

INGREDIENTS
- 20ml/4 tsp neem oil
- 20ml/4 tsp wormwood tincture (pp.18–19)
- 50ml/3 tbs + 1 tsp grapeseed oil

Essential oils:
- 2 drops lemon
- 2 drops orange
- 2 drops grapefruit
- 2 drops cedarwood
- 2 drops eucalyptus
- 2 drops citronella
- 2 drops lavender
- 2 drops sage

MAKES & KEEPS
Makes 90ml/just over ⅓ cup. Keeps 1–2 years.

METHOD
Gently melt the neem oil over a low heat. Mix all the ingredients together and bottle.

Shake before use, then rub it well into fur. In cold weather, warm the mixture gently before applying.

Dogs' Upset Stomach Powder

Courtesy of Barbara Jones

INGREDIENTS
- 30g/1oz dried chamomile, ground
- 60g/2oz dried slippery elm powder

MAKES & KEEPS
Makes 90g/3oz. Keeps 1 year.

METHOD
Mix together well.

Add 1 tsp per 30kg/66lb weight of dog to each meal.

Alternatively, give chamomile powder on its own, 1 tsp with each meal.

Continue use for 1–2 days after symptoms cease.

Chronic Diarrhoea Medicine for Pets

Courtesy of Barbara Jones

Chronic diarrhoea can be a symptom of something more serious, so if it doesn't clear up quickly, see a vet.

INGREDIENTS

Tinctures (pp.18–19):
- 30ml/2 tbs frankincense
- 15ml/1 tbs echinacea
- 20ml/4 tsp golden seal (or baical skullcap)
- 15ml/1 tbs marigold
- 20ml/4 tsp chamomile

MAKES & KEEPS
Makes 100ml/just under ½ cup. Keeps at least 2 years.

METHOD
Mix the tinctures together in a bottle.

Give cats 3–5 drops 3 times daily.

Give dogs 1 tsp for each 30kg/66lb weight of dog 3 times daily.

Pets' Mouth Wash

Courtesy of Barbara Jones

For problem teeth, ulcers and infections.

INGREDIENTS
Tinctures (pp.18–19):
- 30ml/2 tbs marigold (made with a 90% alcohol)
- 30ml/2 tbs echinacea
- 10ml/2 tsp golden seal (or baical skullcap)
- 30ml/2 tbs chamomile

MAKES & KEEPS
Makes 100ml/just under ½ cup.
Keeps 2 years.

METHOD
Mix the tinctures together in a bottle.

Dilute 1 tsp of the liquid in a mug of water, and flush through the pet's mouth with a syringe from side to side. Alternatively, use a sponge to apply to the gums. (Pets don't need to swallow it, though it doesn't hurt them if they do.)

Animal Eye Wash

Courtesy of Barbara Jones

For sticky eyes.

INGREDIENTS
Tinctures (pp.18–19):
- 5ml/1 tsp eyebright
- 5 ml/1 tsp lemon balm
- 5 ml/1 tsp chamomile
- 5 ml/1 tsp golden seal

MAKES & KEEPS
Makes 20ml/4 tsp.
Use immediately.

METHOD
Bathe the eyes 2–3 times daily with ¼ tsp in 50ml/just under ¼ cup cooled boiled water. Make the eye wash fresh each time.

Dogs' Arthritis Medicine

Courtesy of Barbara Jones

INGREDIENTS
Tinctures (pp.18–19):
- 50ml/3 tbs + 1 tsp devil's claw
- 20ml/4 tsp nettle leaf
- 30ml/2 tbs meadowsweet
- 10ml/2 tsp boswelia

MAKES & KEEPS
Makes 100ml/just under ½ cup.
Keeps 2 years.

METHOD
Mix together in a bottle.

Add 1 tsp for each 30kg/66lb weight of dog to food 3 times daily.

> **Caution**
> Treating cats with arthritis is more tricky as salicylates are bad for them. Consult a holistic vet over your cat's arthritis.

Pets' Liver Tonic

Courtesy of Barbara Jones

INGREDIENTS

Tinctures (pp.18–19):
- 30ml/2 tbs milk thistle
- 30ml/2 tbs dandelion root
- 20ml/4 tsp schisandra berry
- 20ml/4 tsp bupleurum root

MAKES & KEEPS

Makes 100ml/just under ½ cup.
Keeps 2 years.

METHOD

Mix together in a bottle.

Give cats 3–5 drops 3 times daily.

Give dogs 1 tsp for each 30kg/66lb weight of dog 3 times daily.

Immune Booster for Horses

Courtesy of Lesley Cunningham

INGREDIENTS

Dried herbs:
- 500g/17oz rubbed nettles
- 500g/17oz clivers
- 500g/17oz marigold flowers
- 500g/17oz dandelion leaves
- 100g/4oz rosehips, chopped
- 100g/4oz burdock root, chopped
- 200g/8oz echinacea roots and tops, chopped

MAKES & KEEPS

A sack of mix to last around 10 weeks.
Keeps 1 year.

METHOD

Place all the ingredients in a large sack. Mix the herbs well.

Add 3 generous handfuls to your horses' feed daily.

Horses' Wart Remedy

Courtesy of Lesley Cunningham

An old recipe for simple warts.

INGREDIENTS
- 1 fresh dandelion root or flower stem

METHOD

Squeeze the milky white dandelion juice on to the wart 2–3 times daily.

Continue use until the wart has gone.

For persistent warts, use together with the Immune Booster for Horses (left).

Horses' Anti-fungal Hoof Paint

Courtesy of Lesley Cunningham

Thrush in horses occurs when the frogs of the hooves become infected.

INGREDIENTS
- 100ml/just under ½ cup of vegetable oil (walnut, grapeseed or sunflower)

Essential oils:
- 50 drops/½ tsp tea tree
- 50 drops/½ tsp lavender

MAKES & KEEPS

Makes 104ml/just under ½ cup, enough for about 20 applications.
Keeps 6 months.

METHOD

Mix the ingredients together in a jar.

Ask a farrier to trim the frogs, removing all dead tissue. Wash the hoof with strong salt water.

Paint the whole area around the frog 2–3 times daily, washing the hoof before each application.

KITCHEN PHARMACY

Sarcoids Cream for Horses

Courtesy of Dedj Leibbrandt

INGREDIENTS
- 100ml/6 tbs + 2 tsp castor oil
- 70g/4 tbs emulsifying wax
- 200ml/¾ cup + 5 tsp chelidonium tea (p.15; make with 1 generous handful of fresh herb in 1 mug of boiling water, infuse for 15 mins with the lid on, then strain)

Tinctures (pp.18–19):
- 50ml/3 tbs + 1 tsp bloodroot
- 50ml/3 tbs + 1 tsp white cedar
- Comfrey Cream for Speedy Healing (p.82)

MAKES & KEEPS
Makes 900g/almost 3¾ cups.
Keeps 1 year.

METHOD
Make the cream using the same method described for Comfrey Cream (p.82). Then mix this cream with an equal amount of Comfrey Cream.

Apply 1–2 times daily. Note: this could take a year to be effective, but it works.

Vitamin E Rich Healing Salve for Animals & People

Courtesy of Lesley Cunningham

INGREDIENTS
- 450ml/just under 2 cups olive oil infused with marigold flowers (p.20)
- 50ml/just under ¼ cup avocado oil
- 50ml/just under ¼ cup vitamin E oil (or another 50ml/just under ¼ cup avocado oil)
- 50g/¼ cup beeswax, grated or broken into small pieces

MAKES & KEEPS
Makes about 600g/2½ cups ointment.
Keeps at least 1 year.

METHOD
Mix the oils and make into a salve with the beeswax (see Solomon's Salves, p.117).

Apply as needed to wounds.

— *Tip* —

THIS HEALING SALVE IS GREAT FOR COWS' UDDERS THAT ARE SORE FROM MASTITIS OR OVER-MILKING. IT'S ALSO HEALING FOR BREAST-FEEDING MOTHERS.

— *Variation* —

FOR SKIN INFECTIONS, ADD 4 HEADS GARLIC CLOVES SEPARATED, PEELED AND CHOPPED, AND INFUSE WITH THE MARIGOLD FLOWERS. THE GARLIC HAS A POWERFUL EXTRA ANTI-INFECTIOUS ACTION.

FOOD & DRINK

There are many lovely things to eat and drink which can either be made with, or incorporate, interesting foraged, grown or bought-in herbs and spices. Nature is bountiful and provides a rich variety of nourishment. In fact wild-growing 'weeds' are the true 'superfoods', being often many times richer in nutrients – especially in essential minerals and vitamins – than their cultivated cousins. In recent years there has been a resurgence of interest in foraging – gathering wild foods from nature. I hope you enjoy exploring foraging, always being mindful to be certain you have gathered what you think you have before eating it. All these recipes are best eaten fresh, but most will keep 1–2 days in airtight containers in the fridge. Here are some ideas to whet your appetite and encourage you to start experimenting…

Probiotic Breakfast

Courtesy of Anne McIntyre

Healthful and healing breakfast for the digestive system.

INGREDIENTS
- 1 large garlic clove
- 2–4 tsp fresh dill leaves
- 1 handful of marigold petals
- 2 tsp fresh oregano
- 3 tsp fresh basil
- 140ml/5oz carton live yogurt
- 2 tbs aloe vera juice

SERVES & KEEPS
Serves 1.
Eat immediately.

METHOD
Add the garlic and fresh herbs to live yogurt daily for breakfast. Alternatively, take 2 tbs aloe vera juice with a little water or ginger tea twice daily.

— *Variation* —

YOU CAN USE ANY OTHER FRESH POT HERBS IF YOU DON'T HAVE THE ONES ABOVE.

Acorn Flour

Courtesy of Anna Richardson

INGREDIENTS
- 4 large handfuls of acorns – discard any with blemishes
- several litres/gallons of water

MAKES & KEEPS
Makes about 2 handfuls of flour.
Keeps 6–12 months if totally dry.

METHOD
Dry the acorns for a couple of days, then remove and discard the shells. Place in a large pan filled with 3–4 times the amount of water to acorns. Boil for about an hour. Strain and discard the water, refill and repeat the process twice more.

Then taste an acorn: if still bitter, boil again. When they are no longer bitter, mash them and leave to cool a little. Strain through a sieve lined with cloth: gather the cloth and squeeze as much water out as possible.

Then spread the mush out on the cloth somewhere warm to dry. This usually takes at least 2 days. Put in a dehumidifier to speed up the process.

Grind it to flour in the coffee grinder and store in a jar. Use as ordinary flour.

Acorn Biscuits

Courtesy of Anna Richardson

INGREDIENTS
- 250g/1 cup butter or margarine
- 250g/¾ cup honey (or 200g/1 cup brown sugar)
- 400g/approx. 3½ cups Acorn Flour (opposite)
- 150g/1 generous cup self-raising flour

MAKES & KEEPS
Makes about 30 biscuits.
Keeps 10–14 days in an airtight container.

METHOD
Preheat the oven to 180°C/350°F/Gas Mark 4.

Melt the butter and honey, then add the other ingredients. Stir and allow to cool until the mixture stiffens up enough to roll into balls (golf-ball size or smaller). Place the balls on a greased baking tray and press down into flat biscuit shapes. Bake in the oven for about 10–15 mins until golden brown. Put on a cooling rack to cool.

> **Caution**
>
> Acorns have been used as food by people everywhere oak trees grow. 0.45kg/1lb of nutritious acorns contains 2,000 calories—but they also contain high levels of tannic acid which makes them unpalatable and toxic to the body, unless they are processed—basically washed a lot—to remove the tannins.

Forest & Corn Goddess Cookies

Courtesy of Sharon Cohen

This recipe prepares the acorns differently to the acorn flour method (opposite).

INGREDIENTS
- 1 handful of chopped acorns (or less if you have harvested fewer)
- 75g/⅓ cup melted butter
- 100ml/⅓ cup + 2 tbs maple tree syrup
- 125ml/½ cup hazelnut milk (at room temperature)
- 125g/½ cup hazelnut meal
- 75g/⅓ cup cornflour

MAKES & KEEPS
Makes around 10–12 cookies.
Keeps 10–14 days in an airtight container.

METHOD
Preheat the oven to 175°C/350°F/Gas Mark 4.

Shell the acorns and soak for a couple of days in 1¼ cups water. Change the water a few times in this period until it remains clear after a couple of hours. Boil the acorns in fresh water for 5–10 mins, then finely chop or chop into small chunks.

Mix the chopped acorns, melted butter and maple syrup.

Make a paste with the hazelnut milk, hazelnut meal and cornflour, then stir this paste into the mixture.

Place small to medium cookie-sized amounts on a greased baking tray. Cook for 12–14 mins, then remove from the oven and leave to cool on the tray.

Plantain Seedy Flapjacks

INGREDIENTS
- 200g/1 cup unsalted butter
- 200g/1 cup brown sugar
- 200g/⅔ cup honey
- 400g/4 cups porridge oats
- 2 tbs plantain seeds (wild-foraged)
- 2 tbs sunflower seeds

MAKES & KEEPS
Makes 16–24.
Keeps 10–14 days in an airtight container.

METHOD
Preheat the oven to 180°C/350°F/Gas Mark 4.

Melt together the butter, sugar and honey, stirring until the sugar is dissolved. Then add the porridge oats and seeds, and mix thoroughly. Put into a 20cm x 30cm/8in x 12in buttered cake tin and bake for 15–20 mins. Score when hot. Leave to cool, then turn out and cut.

Beech Nut Flapjacks

Beech nuts are very small and fiddly to handle – but so nutritious (rich in oils and proteins) that it's worth the effort. Gather plenty of nuts, bring them inside and wait a day or two for the outer shells to open in the warm. Then remove the skin.

INGREDIENTS
- 200g/1 cup unsalted butter
- 200g/1 cup brown sugar
- 200g/⅔ cup honey
- 400g/4 cups porridge oats
- 4 tbs hulled beech nuts (if you can't get enough beech nuts, use 2 tbs beech nuts and 2 tbs chopped walnuts)

MAKES & KEEPS
Makes 16–24.
Keeps 10–14 days in an airtight container.

METHOD
Make as for Plantain Seedy Flapjacks (above), using beech nuts/walnuts in place of plantain/sunflower seeds.

Pharoah's Flapjacks

This recipe is inspired by sacred cakes that the ancient Egyptians offered to their gods.

INGREDIENTS
- 30g/½ cup marsh mallow root (dried or fresh), roughly chopped/shredded
- 60g/½ cup dates, chopped
- 30g/¼ cup almonds, chopped
- 125ml/½ cup water
- 225g/2 sticks butter
- 170g/½ cup honey
- 150g/⅔ cup brown sugar
- 2 tbs sesame seeds
- 30g/½ cup powdered marsh mallow root
- 300g/3 cups porridge oats
- 100g/1 cup quinoa flakes (or oats if preferred)

MAKES & KEEPS
Makes 16–24.
Keeps 10–14 days in an airtight container.

METHOD
Leave the chopped marsh mallow roots, dates and almonds to soak in the water overnight.

Next day, melt the butter together with the honey and sugar. Remove from the heat and stir in the sesame seeds, powdered marsh mallow root, oats and quinoa. Add the soaked marsh mallow, dates and almonds with the water they soaked in.

Bake as for Plantain Seedy Flapjacks (left).

Pine Cookies

Courtesy of Karen Stephenson.

Pine needles are an excellent source of vitamin C.

INGREDIENTS
- 450g/3 cups unbleached flour
- 300g/1½ cups sugar
- 8 tbs pine powder (pine needles, dried and ground to a powder)
- 225g/1 cup melted butter
- 3 eggs/equivalent egg substitute
- 1 tsp vanilla essence

MAKES & KEEPS
Makes 20–30.
Keeps 10–14 days in an airtight container.

METHOD
Preheat the oven to 160°C/325°F/Gas Mark 3.

Place all the dry ingredients into a bowl. In another bowl, blend together the melted butter, eggs and the vanilla. Combine the wet ingredients into the dry ingredients and blend well.

Roll the dough into balls about three-quarters the size of a golf ball. Place on a lightly greased baking tray. Use a fork to flatten the cookies until they are about 5mm/¼in thick. Bake for around 10–12 mins.

Nutty Plantain Snack

Courtesy of Karen Stephenson

INGREDIENTS
- 1 handful of plantain seeds
- 3 handfuls of pumpkin seeds
- 3 handfuls of sesame seeds
- olive oil (enough to just coat the seeds)
- sea salt, to taste

MAKES & KEEPS
Makes 7 handfuls.
Keeps 1–2 weeks in an airtight container.

METHOD
Place the seeds into a bowl, add the olive oil and sea salt. Be sure to coat all the seeds. Either roast the seeds on a baking sheet in an oven (150°C/300°F/Gas Mark 2) for 10–15 mins, or fry in a pan for 5 mins over a medium heat.

Rowanberry Bitters to Stimulate Digestion

INGREDIENTS
- 4 large handfuls of fresh rowanberries
- 250ml/1 cup gin

MAKES & KEEPS
Makes about 500ml/2 cups.
Keeps 2–3 years.

METHOD
Squeeze the juice from the rowanberries using a juicer. Mix well with the gin. If you don't have a juicer, liquidize the berries and gin together in a blender and strain through a mesh strainer. Repeat the straining but through muslin.

Take 5–10 drops in a little water before meals to stimulate digestion, as required.

Savoury Pancakes

Buckwheat contains rutin which strengthens the blood vessels. This recipe adds in circulation-boosting herbs and is particularly good for rebuilding veins. It also tastes great!

INGREDIENTS

- 180g/1 cup raw buckwheat, measured then ground
- ¼ tsp salt
- 250ml/1 cup water
- 2 tsp dried rosemary, ground
- 1–2 dried horse chestnut seeds (conkers), ground – do not use more than this (optional)
- ¼ tsp cayenne pepper or paprika
- coconut oil or butter, for frying

SERVES & KEEPS

Serves 2–4. Serve hot straight from the pan. The batter will keep uncooked in the fridge and can be cooked the next day.

METHOD

Make a batter by mixing the buckwheat, salt and water and beating to a smooth batter. Leave to stand for ½–2 hours.

Add the rosemary, horse chestnut seeds (if using) and cayenne pepper. Beat the mixture again, then heat a little oil/butter in a frying pan and cook for about 10 minutes on a low heat, until browned. Buckwheat pancakes cook more slowly than wheat pancakes – be patient and cook them until they look just right.

Buckwheat Blinis

Courtesy of Sucandra Devi dasi

These sweet mini-pancakes are circulation-boosters. Serve with Many Berry Cordial (p.55) for an extra boost, as blood vessels are helped by the flavonoids found in all red fruits.

INGREDIENTS

- 180g/1 cup raw buckwheat, measured then ground
- ¼ tsp salt
- 250ml/1 cup water
- 1 tsp ground cinnamon
- 1 tsp ground ginger

SERVES & KEEPS

Serves 2–4. Serve hot straight from the pan. The batter will keep uncooked in the fridge and can be cooked the next day.

METHOD

Make a batter with the buckwheat, salt, water and spices. Beat and proceed as for Savoury Pancakes (left).

FRITTERS, PAKORAS & TEMPURA

The following fritters, pakoras and tempura are made with a gluten-free batter made from gram (chickpea) flour.

Make a batter by mixing 100g/1 cup of the flour with a little water, so that the paste has the texture of thick custard. Leave to stand for 10–30 mins.

Gram (chickpea) flour is a nourishing fibre-rich food containing some healthy amino acids and minerals, and is low in sodium and fats.

Elderflower Fritters

Courtesy of Wizz Holland

INGREDIENTS
- 6–7 heads freshly picked elderflowers
- 100g/1 cup gram (chickpea) flour batter (see main intro recipe)
- sunflower oil, for frying
- caster sugar, to taste

MAKES & KEEPS
Makes 6–7 fritters.
Keeps 2 days in the fridge.

METHOD
De-insect the heads of elderflowers by placing in a paper bag scrunched up at the top for an hour (this allows insects to vacate!) and then remove from the bag, shaking gently. Dip fresh flower heads into the batter, holding them by the stalk, and deep-fry for 2–5 mins.

When golden brown, remove from the oil and drain on kitchen paper. Sprinkle with caster sugar.

Comfrey Fritters

Packed with minerals and vitamins, these can also be made with borage leaves.

INGREDIENTS
- 100g/1 cup gram (chickpea) flour batter (see main intro recipe)
- sweet version: ½ tsp ground cinnamon or nutmeg; sunflower oil, for frying
- savoury version: ¼ tsp asafoetida; sesame oil, for frying
- 8–10 freshly picked young comfrey leaves

MAKES & KEEPS
Makes 8–10.
Keeps 2 days in the fridge.

METHOD
Add either savoury or sweet spices to the batter. Wipe the comfrey leaves through it, then deep-fry them for 1 min in sunflower/sesame oil, depending on your chosen version. Drain and serve.

Pungent Pakoras

INGREDIENTS
- 100g/1 cup gram (chickpea) flour batter (see main intro recipe)
- 1 handful of fresh wild garlic, chopped (or garlic mustard)
- 1 medium potato, chopped
- oil, for frying
- salt and pepper, to taste

MAKES & KEEPS
Makes 8–12.
Keeps 2 days in the fridge.

METHOD
Mix the ingredients together. Drop a ball of the mixture into hot oil and deep-fry for 1–2 mins or until golden brown. Drain and serve hot.

Pennywort Sattvic Tempura

INGREDIENTS
- 100g/1 cup gram (chickpea) flour batter (see main intro recipe)
- ½ tsp wasabi powder (or ground dried horseradish root)
- 1 generous handful of pennywort leaves (or other edible greens, see p.154, Mess of Greens)
- coconut or sesame oil, for frying
- tamari/soy sauce, to taste

MAKES & KEEPS
Makes 8–12.
Keeps 2 days in the fridge.

METHOD
Add the wasabi or horseradish to the batter, dip the pennywort leaves in it and fry for 1–2 mins until golden brown.

Drain and serve with tamari (soy sauce).

Lamb's Quarters Herbal Salt

Courtesy of Karen Stephenson

Lamb's quarters, like most other wild green herbs, is very rich in vitamins and minerals. This is a salt that provides for many of the body's mineral needs.

INGREDIENTS

Dried herbs:
- 4 tbs dulce (or any other available seaweed)
- 2 tbs lamb's quarters leaves
- 2 tbs thyme or rosemary
- 2 tbs dill
- 2 tbs marjoram or oregano

MAKES & KEEPS
Makes 100g/1 cup.
Keeps 3–6 months in an airtight jar.

METHOD
Gently toast the dulce using a skillet or heavy frying pan for a few minutes until very crisp.

Grind the lamb's quarters leaves and herbs in a blender or a coffee mill while the seaweed cools. Then grind the dulce and combine with ground herbs. Store in a shaker, and use as you would table salt.

Herb Salt

INGREDIENTS
- 100g/½ cup coarse sea salt
- 3 tbs fresh rosemary leaves, removed from stems
- 3 tbs fresh thyme leaves, removed from stems
- 3 tbs fresh marjoram leaves
- 200g/1 cup sea salt (kosher salt is ideal)

MAKES & KEEPS
Makes 350g/2 cups.
Keeps 6–12 months in an airtight jar.

METHOD
Put the 100g/½ cup coarse salt and herbs in a blender and pulse-blend to grind until well mixed (but not ground to a powder). Then add the sea salt and pulse a few times to mix well in.

Spread out to dry on a tray, and cover with a tea towel. Leave to dry for 2–3 hours. Sprinkle on raw cucumber for a tasty snack.

Wild Herb Savoury Cream

INGREDIENTS
- 120g/1 cup raw cashew nuts
- water, to soak
- 125ml/½ cup water
- 4 tbs mixed fresh herbs, e.g. thyme, sage, marjoram, wild garlic: make your own mixture from what is available
- 1 tsp miso
- juice of ½ lemon (optional)
- pinch of salt, to taste (optional)

MAKES & KEEPS
Makes 150g/1 cup.
Keeps 3 days in the fridge.

METHOD
Soak the cashew nuts for 3–7 hours in water. Drain them and blend until smooth with the other ingredients.

Serve with crackers, or use as a spread on bread.

Rose & Cashew Cream

A lovely alternative to dairy cream to serve with pancakes.

INGREDIENTS
- 120g/1 cup raw cashews
- water, to soak
- 125ml/½ cup rosewater
- 1 tsp stevia powder
- ¼ tsp cardamom powder (optional)

MAKES & KEEPS
Makes 150g/1 cup.
Keeps 3 days in the fridge.

METHOD
Soak the cashews for 3–7 hours in water. Drain and blend until smooth with the rosewater, stevia and cardamom.

Sweet Flower Sandwiches

A lovely feast for a children's tea party.

INGREDIENTS
- 4 slices of white bread
- butter and granulated sugar, to taste
- 1 handful of fresh clover flowers

MAKES & KEEPS
Makes 2 rounds.
Eat the same day.

METHOD
Make the sandwiches by putting the flowers on freshly buttered bread with a little sugar sprinkled on. As an alternative, try making these with primroses or violets.

Ivy-leaved Toadflax Sandwiches

INGREDIENTS
- small handful of ivy-leaved toadflax leaves and flowers
- 4 slices rye or granary bread
- butter, salad cream/mayonnaise, and salt and pepper, to taste

MAKES & KEEPS
Makes 2 rounds.
Eat the same day.

METHOD
Place the ivy-leaf on freshly buttered and dressed bread. Add salt and pepper to taste. You can also make these with jack by the hedge/garlic mustard and plantain.

Pennywort Sandwiches

INGREDIENTS
- 1 handful of pennywort leaves, freshly picked and chopped
- 1 tsp olive oil
- 1 avocado, mashed
- 1 tsp lime juice
- salt and black pepper, to taste
- 4 slices granary bread, lightly toasted

MAKES & KEEPS
Makes 2 rounds.
Eat the same day.

METHOD
Mix the pennywort with the olive oil, avocado and lime juice. Add salt and pepper to taste. Spoon the mixture on to the bread to make a sandwich. Enjoy!

Fennel Oatcakes

Adapted from a recipe by Susun Weed

INGREDIENTS
- 500g/2 cups rolled oats
- ½ tsp baking powder
- ½ tsp salt
- 250g/1 cup oatmeal
- 2 tsp fennel seeds
- 2 tbs olive oil or melted organic butter
- 90–120ml/6–8 tbs hot water
- 125g/½ cup rolled oats, for rolling

MAKES & KEEPS
Makes 24–32.
Keeps 10–14 days in an airtight container.

METHOD
Grind the 500g/2 cups of rolled oats to a fine meal in a blender or grinder – you'll get about 375g/1½ cups of meal. Mix this with the baking powder, salt, oatmeal, fennel and oil or butter.

Add just enough hot water to form a ball of dough. Divide into 2. Sprinkle a few oats on your work surface and roll out each ball (adding more oats as needed) to 2 handspans wide (about 23cm/9in in diameter).

Cut each circle into 6–8 wedges. Cook on a baking tray at 180°C/350°F/Gas Mark 4 for 15 mins, or in a cast-iron skillet or heavy frying pan for 8 mins a side.

FOOD & DRINK

Rosemary & Poppy Seed Oatcakes

Adapted from a recipe by Susun Weed

INGREDIENTS
- 500g/2 cups rolled oats
- ½ tsp baking powder
- ½ tsp salt
- 250g/1 cup oatmeal
- 2 tsp dried rosemary, rubbed small
- 2 tsp poppy seeds
- 2 tbs olive oil or melted organic butter
- 90–120ml/6–8 tbs hot water
- 125g/½ cup rolled oats, for rolling

MAKES & KEEPS
Makes 24–32.
Keeps 10–14 days in an airtight container.

METHOD
Make as for Fennel Oatcakes (opposite), adding the rosemary and poppy seeds in place of the fennel seeds.

Yellow Dock Crackers

Courtesy of Karen Stephenson

INGREDIENTS
- 1 handful of yellow dock seed, crushed
- 150g/1 cup flour of your choice
- 1 tsp sea salt

MAKES & KEEPS
Makes 15–30 crackers.
Keeps 10–14 days in an airtight container.

METHOD
Preheat the oven to 190°C/375°F/Gas Mark 5.

Mix together the crushed yellow dock seed, flour and salt in a bowl. Very gradually add a little water until the dough is pliable (not sticky).

Roll the dough thinly on a well-floured work surface, and cut into desired shapes.

Transfer them on to a well-greased baking sheet, and bake for 10–12 mins, or until crisp.

> *When you harvest yellow dock seeds for this recipe, they must be brown. Remove all leaves, stems or anything else to ensure you have only the seeds. Store whole seeds in a paper bag. Once ground, store in an airtight jar.*

Anti-flu Soup

INGREDIENTS
- 500ml/2 cups vegetable broth (see Method)
- 3–4 spring onions or leeks, chopped
- 2 tbs coconut oil
- 2 tbs flour
- 1 stalk lemongrass, very finely chopped
- 2 handfuls of wild greens (or spinach), chopped
- 500ml/2 cups coconut milk

SERVES & KEEPS
Serves 1–2.
Keeps 2 days in the fridge. Thoroughly reheat before eating.

METHOD
Make your vegetable broth by simmering a selection of vegetables in water with salt and pepper for 1 hour. Strain and keep the liquid.

Place the onions or leeks and coconut oil in a large saucepan and sauté on a low heat for 5 mins. Add the flour and continue to stir over the heat for 1–3 mins until thick.

Add the broth, lemongrass and greens, then allow to simmer for 15 mins. Add the coconut milk, then simmer for a further 5 mins.

Sinus-clearing Soup

Courtesy of Sue Wine

INGREDIENTS
- 1 litre/1 quart water
- 115g/1 cup sliced celery
- 140g/1 cup thinly sliced carrots
- 2 large handfuls of fresh parsley or other green herb
- 2–3 whole green or red hot chillies
- 1 head garlic, cloves separated, peeled and crushed
- 2 tsp miso

MAKES & KEEPS
Serves 1–2.
Keeps 2 days in the fridge. Thoroughly reheat before eating.

METHOD
Add all the ingredients except the garlic and miso to a large saucepan. Cover with a lid, bring to the boil and simmer for 25 mins. Then add the crushed garlic and cook for a further 5 mins, before stirring in the miso and serving.

Nettle & Wild Garlic Lentil Soup

This delicious and nourishing, mineral-rich soup is adapted from a recipe in Kitchen of Love (2013). If you can't get the nettles and ramsons, use other wild or cultivated edible greens.

INGREDIENTS
- 190g/1 cup brown lentils
- 1.44 litres/6 cups water
- 3 tbs olive oil
- ½ tsp ground black pepper
- 1 tsp asafoetida, powdered
- 150g/1 cup potatoes, cubed
- 115g/1 cup celery, diced, with leaves
- 1 large handful of fresh nettle tops, chopped (wear gloves!)
- 1 large handful of freshly picked ramsons (wild garlic), chopped
- ½ roasted red pepper, cut into julienne strips
- 1 tsp ground coriander
- 1 tsp ground cumin
- 2 tbs fresh lemon juice
- 1–1½ tsp salt, to taste
- 7g/¼ cup each parsley and coriander leaves, very finely chopped

MAKES & KEEPS
Serves 4.
Keeps 2 days in the fridge. Thoroughly reheat before eating.

METHOD
Bring the water and lentils to the boil. Simmer for 15 mins, or until the lentils start to break up.

Warm the oil in another pan. Add the black pepper and asafoetida to the potatoes and stir-fry over a medium heat. After 2–3 mins add the celery. Fry for another minute, then add to the simmering lentils.

Cook for a further 20 mins, then add the nettles, ramsons and all the other ingredients except the salt, parsley and coriander leaves. Cook for 5–10 mins.

Add the salt, parsley and coriander. Serve with bread or rice.

Nature's Bounty

These wild plants can be foraged and eaten raw or cooked (with greens, salads, stir-fries and more).

- hawthorn leaves and blossom
- lime flower leaves
- dandelion
- jack by the hedge
- garlic mustard
- wood sorrel
- sheep sorrel
- ox-eye daisy leaves
- chickweed
- daisy leaves and flowers
- plantain leaves
- primrose flowers
- clover leaves and flowers
- rosebay
- purslane
- bramble leaf buds
- pennywort
- violet leaves and flowers

THE RECIPES

Wild Garlic Bread

INGREDIENTS
- 1 handful of fresh wild garlic, chopped
- 240g/1 cup butter
- pinch of salt
- 1 loaf of rustic bread

MAKES & KEEPS
Makes 1 loaf.
Eat immediately.

METHOD
Preheat the oven to 175°C/350°F/Gas Mark 4.

Blend the chopped wild garlic, butter and salt together well. Make diagonal cuts along the loaf – just partway through – about 3cm/1¼in apart. Spread the herb butter between each slice.

Wrap the whole loaf in foil and place in the oven for 15–20 mins.

Nature Smoothie

Courtesy of Shelley Harrison

This green smoothie is a mineral-rich boost that comes straight from nature.

INGREDIENTS
- 1 cucumber
- 1 avocado
- 1 handful of a mix of 2 or more of chickweed, dandelion leaves, nettles, nasturtiums, plantain, garlic mustard or other edible greens
- 500ml/2 cups water

SERVES & KEEPS
Serves 2–3.
Drink immediately.

METHOD
Whizz everything together in a blender and serve.

Wild Garlic Pesto

Courtesy of Annie Gardner

INGREDIENTS
- 70g/½ cup sunflower seeds (or cashews or pine nuts), soaked overnight in water
- 1 tbs umaboshi plum seasoning
- 4–6 leaves of wild garlic (or ½ handful of garlic mustard leaves)
- 2 tbs olive oil
- 4 tbs water
- 1 handful of wild greens e.g. chickweed, dandelion leaves, nettles or spinach

MAKES & KEEPS
Makes approx. 250ml/1 cup.
Eat the same day.

METHOD
Strain and rinse the soaked seeds/nuts. Blend with the other ingredients until you reach the consistency you desire. Add more water if it is too thick.

Serve with pasta, baked sweet potatoes or quinoa with steamed vegetables or salad. Also spread on oatcakes or bread.

Herb Pesto

INGREDIENTS
- 70g/½ cup pine nuts, soaked overnight in water
- few sprigs fresh rosemary leaves, stalks removed
- few sprigs fresh oregano
- few sprigs parsley
- 1 tsp asafoetida
- 2 tbs olive oil
- 4 tbs water
- 1 handful of wild greens e.g. chickweed, dandelion leaves, nettles (or spinach)

MAKES & KEEPS
Makes approx. 250ml/1 cup.
Keeps 2 days in the fridge.

METHOD
Make as for Wild Garlic Pesto (above).

Calcium-rich Herb Salad

Courtesy of Anne McIntyre

All of these nutritious herbs are rich in minerals, particularly calcium vital for keeping your bones strong. The fiery rocket and nasturtium as well as the aromatic dill, coriander and parsley leaves will promote digestion and absorption, ensuring that these vital nutrients reach your bones.

INGREDIENTS
- nasturtium flowers and leaves
- tender young plantain leaves
- young dandelion leaves
- borage flowers and leaves
- rocket
- parsley
- coriander
- dill
- mint
- marigold flowers

KEEPS
Keeps 2 days in the fridge.

METHOD
Pick fresh any or all of these delicious salad herbs. Serve with a simple dressing made with olive oil and herbal vinegar.

Chickweed Sag Paneer

Adapted from a recipe in Kitchen of Love *(2013).*

INGREDIENTS
- 2 tbs ghee or sesame oil
- 1½ tsp cumin seeds
- 1 green chilli, seeded and very finely chopped
- 1 tbs fresh root ginger, chopped
- 1 tsp asafoetida
- 1 tsp ground coriander
- 1 tsp ground cumin
- 1 tsp garam masala
- 1 tsp ground turmeric
- 600g/3½–4 cups tomatoes, roughly blended
- 1 tsp flour
- 900g/10 cups chopped spinach (will shrink when cooked), lightly cooked
- 2 handfuls of/2 cups fresh chickweed, roughly chopped and cooked
- 2 tbs crème fraîche
- 350g/12oz paneer, cubed and fried to a light gold colour then put into lightly salted water

SERVES & KEEPS
Serves 4–6.
Keeps 2 days in the fridge.

METHOD
Gently heat the ghee or oil for a few minutes and add the cumin seeds. Add the chilli and ginger and turn the heat down. Add all the ground spices, stir for a few minutes and add the puréed tomatoes.

Mix the flour and a dash of water to a smooth paste in a small dish and add to the pan, stirring and cooking for a few minutes. Add the cooked spinach and chickweed, and stir for a couple of mins.

Add the crème fraîche and mix in well. Drain the paneer from the salt water and add to the rest, simmering gently for 5 mins.

Serve with rice and poppadoms.

Mess of Greens

To get the modern palette used to wild greens, try this recipe.

INGREDIENTS
- 500g/6 cups dark green cabbage or kale leaves, loosely chopped
- 4–5 heads of fresh yarrow flowers, finely chopped
- around 8–10 fresh nettle tops (gathered with gloves and cut up with scissors)
- 1 handful of fresh ground elder, finely chopped

SERVES & KEEPS
Serves 2–4.
Keeps 2 days in the fridge.

METHOD
Mix the greens and steam lightly for 4–5 mins.

To serve, pour on a little olive oil and the herb vinegar of your choice.

Cattail Rice Recipe

Courtesy of Karen Stephenson

INGREDIENTS
- 1 tbs olive oil
- ½ handful of cattail shoots, peeled and chopped
- 4–6/1 cup chopped shallots
- 2 garlic cloves, chopped
- 600g/3 cups cooked brown rice
- 2 tbs tamari
- ½ tsp cayenne pepper

SERVES & KEEPS
Serves 2–4.
Keeps 2 days in the fridge.

METHOD
Heat the olive oil in a large skillet or heavy frying pan. Add the cattail shoots, shallots and garlic and sauté for 5 mins. Add the remaining ingredients and cook until the rice is hot. Stir frequently to prevent sticking.

Gobō – Burdock Roots Japanese-style

Courtesy of Louise Berliner

INGREDIENTS
- 1 tbs sesame oil
- 1–2 burdock roots, cut into matchstick-sized pieces
- 2 medium carrots, cut into matchstick-sized pieces
- 1–2 tbs rice wine or Gorse Wine (p.177) (optional)
- 2 tsp tamari
- 2.5cm/1in piece fresh root ginger, grated
- 1–2 tsp toasted sesame seeds

SERVES & KEEPS
Serves 2.
Keeps 2 days in the fridge.

METHOD
Heat the oil and sauté the burdock root until covered in oil. Layer the carrots on the top, and add a little water (and/or wine if using) to just cover the burdock.

Cover with a lid and cook over a medium-low heat for 10–15 mins. Add the tamari and simmer away the liquid. Once the liquid has almost simmered away, add the ginger, toss and add the toasted sesame seeds.

Buttered Burdock Stems

INGREDIENTS
- 2 handfuls of burdock stems
- butter and herb salt and pepper, to taste

SERVES & KEEPS
Serves 4–6.
Keeps 2 days in the fridge.

METHOD
Choose young plants and cut stems close to the ground. Cut the leaves away. Wearing gloves (they will stain your hands), peel away the greyish covering skin on the stems to reveal bright green inner stems.

Steam the burdock in a steamer for 6–10 mins until tender. Serve hot with butter, herb salt and pepper. Alternatively, eat the stems cold, chopped up and drizzled with a herbal vinegar (pp.163–65).

Roasted Reed Rhizomes

Courtesy of Karen Stephenson

A delicious foraged meal.

INGREDIENTS
- 12 reed (Phragmites) rhizomes (at least 15cm/6in in length)
- 2–3 tbs olive oil
- sea salt and pepper (or nutmeg if preferred), to taste

SERVES & KEEPS
Serves 4.
Keeps 2 days in the fridge.

METHOD
After washing the Phragmites rhizomes, coat them with olive oil and spices.

Place on a baking sheet. Bake at 175°C/350°F/Gas Mark 4 for 25 mins.

Angelica Supreme

This is a delicious Icelandic speciality. Angelica roots and stems are also good to eat raw — try them with a dip.

INGREDIENTS
- 1 handful of young angelica stalks, freshly picked
- 25g/2 tbs butter (plus a little extra)
- 25g/2 tbs plain flour
- 550ml/2¼ cups milk
- salt and pepper, to taste

SERVES & KEEPS
Serves 1–2.
Keeps 2 days in the fridge.

METHOD
Prepare the stems as for Buttered Burdock Stems (left), either steaming or boiling until soft. Put a knob of butter on them and place in a casserole dish.

Make a white sauce by gently melting the butter and stirring in the flour, and cooking for 1–2 minutes. Gradually add the milk, a tiny bit at a time, stirring all the time and cooking for about 8 mins to make a sauce with the consistency of custard. Add salt and pepper.

Pour over the angelica stems. Bake for 10–15 mins in a warm oven.

Hot Oil

This versatile oil can be used in cooking to spice up dishes, or as a lotion for aching muscles.

INGREDIENTS
- 250ml/1 cup olive oil
- 30g/¼ cup cayenne pepper
- 30g/¼ cup ground ginger

MAKES & KEEPS
Makes 250ml/1 cup. Keeps 1 year.

METHOD
Make as for an infused oil (p.20).

Wild Greens

INGREDIENTS
- 1 generous handful of fresh kale or spinach or other greens, shredded
- 1 handful of chickweed
- 4–5 fresh borage leaves (if available)
- 1 small handful of fresh violet leaves and flowers
- knob of butter or olive oil
- pinch of nutmeg and herb salt (to taste)

SERVES & KEEPS
Serves 2–4.
Eat same day.

METHOD
In a steamer, lightly steam the kale for 3 mins. Add the chickweed, borage and violet leaves and cook for a further 2 mins.

Serve with a knob of butter and a little herb salt.

Wild Toothwort Sauce

Courtesy of Karen Stephenson

Toothwort is milder and a tiny bit sweeter than horseradish. Try this dip with chips or with Yellow Dock Crackers (p.149).

INGREDIENTS
- 3 tbs toothwort root, finely chopped
- 2 tbs soured cream
- 3 tbs mayonnaise or egg-free substitute
- cracked pepper, to taste
- ¼ tsp cayenne pepper (or less if you wish)

MAKES & KEEPS
Makes 100g/½ cup.
Keeps up to 4 weeks in the fridge.

METHOD
Simply combine all the ingredients in a mixing bowl and blend well.

Hot Cayenne Tincture for Chilli Hot Chocolate & More

Use 5–20 drops of this fiery tincture to spice up a drink or a dish.

This is known as 'capsicum forte' because it is seriously strong. Cayenne is a good addition to many medicines, because it stimulates the circulation and helps with absorption of herbs.

INGREDIENTS
- 75g/¾ cup cayenne pepper
- 500ml/2 cups organic vodka

MAKES & KEEPS
Makes 500ml/2 cups.
Keeps indefinitely.

METHOD
Make as for tinctures (pp.18–19) and store in a dropper bottle. Care is needed: wear gloves when straining and do not get this tincture in your eyes.

Add around 10 drops to a mug of hot chocolate, to taste.

Experiment with how much to add to cooking, according to taste.

As a warming and stimulating medicine, take 5–20 drops in a mug of warm water.

Horseradish Sauce

This makes a traditional and strong sauce.

INGREDIENTS
- 3 tbs fresh grated horseradish root
- 2 tbs soured cream
- 3 tbs mayonnaise or egg-free substitute
- Cracked pepper, to taste

MAKES & KEEPS
Makes around 125ml/½ cup.
Keeps up to 4 weeks in the fridge.

METHOD
Combine all the ingredients in a mixing bowl and blend well.

Red Clover Syrup

Full of calcium and other minerals, this absolutely delicious syrup is gorgeous with pancakes – and also is medicinal.

INGREDIENTS
- 325ml/1¼ cups water
- 600g/3 cups white sugar
- 2 handfuls of fresh red clover flowers

MAKES & KEEPS
Makes approx. 900ml/30fl.oz.
Keeps up to a year until opened, then up to 1 month in the fridge.

METHOD
Make the syrup (pp.21–22) by boiling the water and sugar briskly for 3 mins. Then pour the plain syrup over the flowers in a bowl and leave to stand for 1–2 hours until cool. Strain and bottle.

Hawthorn Flower Syrup

Courtesy of Lucy Wells

Hawthorn flowers make a tasty syrup that preserves their heart-strengthening and uplifting qualities.

INGREDIENTS
- 325ml/1¼ cups water
- 600g/3 cups white sugar
- 7 tbs rosewater
- 50ml/¼ cup lemon juice
- 2 good handfuls of freshly picked hawthorn flowers, twigs removed

MAKES & KEEPS
Makes approx. 900ml/30fl.oz.
Keeps up to a year until opened, then up to 1 month in the fridge.

METHOD
Make the syrup (pp.21–22) by boiling the water and sugar briskly for 3 mins. Mix the rosewater and lemon juice with the syrup. Then pour over the flowers in a bowl and leave to stand for 1–2 hours until cool. Strain and bottle.

Forsythia Syrup

Courtesy of Karen Stephenson

Capture the joyous yellow of forsythia with this tasty syrup.

INGREDIENTS
- 750ml/3 cups water
- 600g/3 cups white sugar
- 3 handfuls of fresh forsythia flowers, rinsed

MAKES & KEEPS
Makes 1 litre/1 quart.
Keeps 3 months in the fridge.

METHOD
Make the syrup (pp.21–22) by boiling the water and sugar briskly for 3 mins. Then pour the plain syrup over the flowers in a bowl and leave to stand for 1–2 hours until cool. Strain and bottle.

Queen Anne's Lace Jelly

Courtesy of Karen Stephenson

INGREDIENTS
- 2 handfuls of fresh Queen Anne's lace flowers
- 1 litre/1 quart boiling water
- 4 tbs lemon juice
- 50g/2oz pack powdered pectin
- 800g/3½ cups + 2 tbs white sugar

MAKES & KEEPS
Makes 1.5kg/around 3lb (5 x 300g/10oz jars). Well-preserved jam keeps for years. Best to use within 1 year.

METHOD
Steep the flowers in the water, covered, for 30 mins, then strain. Measure 750ml/3 cups of the liquid into a pot. Add the lemon juice and pectin. Bring to a rolling boil, stirring constantly. Add the sugar and continue to stir.

Cook and stir until the mixture comes to a rolling boil, then boil for 1 further minute. Remove from the heat.

Skim the scum off the top and discard. Pour into sterilized jars leaving 5mm/¼in free at the top. Sterilize the loosely sealed jars for a further 5 mins.

Spiced Hawthorn & Rowan Berry Jelly

Full of vitamin C, this is delicious on oatcakes or with savoury dishes.

INGREDIENTS
- 1kg/2lb rowan berries, stalks removed
- 1kg/2lb hawthorn berries, stalks removed
- 1kg/2lb crab apples, halved
- 2 cinnamon sticks, broken up
- 6 cloves (optional)
- water and sugar (variable quantity)

MAKES & KEEPS
Makes up to 5kg/11lb of jelly. Keeps 1–2 years.

METHOD
Put the berries and apples together with the spices in a large pan, adding enough water to cover. Bring to the boil, then simmer for 30 mins. Mash and leave to cool for 1–2 hours.

Pour into a double layer of muslin (or jelly bag if you have one) and leave overnight to drip through slowly. In the morning measure your liquid, then pour into a saucepan and bring to the boil. For every 600g/2½ cups of decoction add 400g/2 cups of sugar and then bring to the boil again.

Boil for 1 further min, then remove from the heat. Prepare and jar your jelly as for Queen Anne's Lace Jelly (left).

Spicy Elder & Bilberry Rob

A rob is a fruit syrup that is boiled down to a thick paste, sometimes made without added sugar when using naturally sugar-rich fruit. Add hot water to make it into a lovely hot drink — not only tasty but also an immune-boosting tonic and a cold and flu remedy.

INGREDIENTS
- several heads/4 cups fresh elderberries, stripped from the stalks/stems
- 150g/1 cup bilberries or blueberries
- 250ml/1 cup water
- 2 cinnamon sticks
- 8 cloves
- ½ nutmeg, grated
- up to 225g/1 cup sugar (variable)

MAKES & KEEPS
Makes approx. 200g/around 1 cup.
Keeps up to a year before opening if made well and stored in sterilized jars. Keep in the fridge and use each jar within 3–4 weeks once opened.

METHOD
Bring the berries to the boil with the water, then cover with a lid and simmer for 2 hours. Mash the mixture well, then press out thoroughly through muslin. (Wear gloves if you don't want purple hands!) Add the spices and 200g/1 cup sugar for every 500ml/2 cups of juice. Return to the heat and simmer for 40 mins. Strain with a sieve or strainer and pour into sterilized jars.

Take a generous spoonful daily or more often to protect against colds and flu.

Radharani's Favourite Ice Cream

A simple and delicious ice cream, fit for a goddess.

INGREDIENTS
- 250g/1 cup double cream
- 120ml/½ cup Elderflower Cordial (p.162, or Hawthorn Flower Syrup or Red Clover Syrup, p.157)
- 250g/1 cup condensed milk

MAKES & KEEPS
Makes 8–12 servings.
Keeps 1 month in the freezer.

METHOD
Beat the cream for 1–2 mins, then mix with the elderflower cordial and condensed milk.

Put into a freezeproof container then freeze. It should be ready in about 2–3 hours.

After-dinner Mouth Freshener

Similar recipes are known in India as Mukhwas ('mouth freshener').

INGREDIENTS
Dried seeds:
- 2 tsp aniseed
- 2 tsp fennel
- 2 tsp lovage
- 2 drops peppermint essential oil

MAKES & KEEPS
Makes 6 tbs.
Keeps 6–12 months.

METHOD
Mix the seeds together and sprinkle with peppermint oil. Shake well and store in an airtight container.

Chew a sprinkle of seeds after a meal.

Sweet Pickled Purslane Stems

Courtesy of Karen Stephenson

INGREDIENTS
- 60g/¼ cup fine sea salt
- 1 litre/1 quart ice-cold water
- 3–4 handfuls of fresh purslane stems, washed and removed from leaves (the leaves can be eaten)
- 2 large onions
- 375ml/1½ cups Apple Cider Vinegar (p.165)
- 400g/2 cups cane sugar
- 1 tbs mustard seeds
- ½ tsp turmeric powder
- 250ml/1 cup water

MAKES & KEEPS
Makes 3–4 500g/½ quart jars.
Keeps in the fridge for 6 months.

METHOD
Mix the salt and iced water, and place the purslane and onions into it for 1–2 hours in the fridge.

Heat the remaining ingredients to boiling point, stirring occasionally. Add the drained purslane and onions, and boil for 5 mins. Leave to cool for 30–60 mins.

Spoon the onions and purslane into preserving jars using a slotted spoon, then pour in the juice to fill each jar.

Pickled Ginger

Pickle lovers will eat these on their own, or with sushi — or with any meal!

INGREDIENTS
- 200g/2 cups thinly sliced fresh root ginger
- 2 litres/2 quarts boiling water
- 500ml/2 cups rice or white vinegar
- 150g/¾ cup caster sugar
- 1 tbs salt
- 1 nutmeg, grated (optional)

MAKES & KEEPS
Makes almost 900ml/30fl.oz.
Keeps in the fridge for up to 6 months.

METHOD
Drop the ginger into the boiling water and leave it for 3 mins. Drain it well and place in a sterilized 1 litre/1 quart jar (p.17).

Heat together the vinegar, sugar, salt and nutmeg, if using, and boil for 5 mins. Pour over the ginger slices, put the lid on and leave to cool overnight before refrigerating. This is ready to eat the next day.

Marsh Mallow Sweetmeats

Nothing like the modern version, full of glucose and gelatine, these rich sweets can also calm and heal the stomach and the lungs.

INGREDIENTS
- approx. 2½ tbs honey
- 25g/1oz dried marsh mallow root, powdered

MAKES & KEEPS
Makes 14–20 sweets.
Keeps 1–2 months in an airtight container.

METHOD
Warm the honey and mix in the root to make a stiff paste. Roll into balls and leave to cool.

— *Tip* —

IF YOU PUT A LITTLE ALMOND OIL ON YOUR FINGERS BEFORE ROLLING THE SWEETMEATS, IT STOPS THEM STICKING.

Elecampane Sweets

These delicious sweets also help the digestion and the lungs.

INGREDIENTS
- 2½ tbs honey
- 25g/1oz dried elecampane root, powdered

MAKES & KEEPS
Makes 14–20 sweets.
Keeps 1–2 months in an airtight container.

METHOD
Make and store in the same way as marsh mallow sweetmeats (above).

Pure Liquorice

For liquorice lovers, a method of making pure solid liquorice.

INGREDIENTS
- 500g/18oz dried liquorice, roughly chopped
- 5 litres/1 gallon water

MAKES & KEEPS
Makes about 200g/7oz solid liquorice extract. Keeps indefinitely.

METHOD
Decoct the liquorice in the water (p.15), simmering covered for 30 mins. Strain well through muslin.

Heat the decocted liquid in a double boiler or bain-marie, letting the water evaporate off until the liquorice extract becomes more and more concentrated. After 1½ hours, you will be left with an almost solid, sticky black goo.

Put the mixture into moulds or flat on a greased/lined tray. Leave it to continue drying out for about 2 weeks (though in warm climates, or if you use a dehumidifier, this can take only 5 days). Once your liquorice has dried (it will become solid), cut into pieces. You can eat it as sweets or dissolve in water to use in other recipes.

Caution
For some, eating excessive amounts of licorice can raise the blood pressure and cause oedema (water retention), so don't regularly eat more than 1–2 small pieces daily. Diabetics should be aware that licorice is very high in sugar.

Crystallized Ginger

INGREDIENTS
- 450g/4½ cups fresh sliced root ginger
- 1.5 litres/5 cups water
- 400g/2 cups caster sugar

MAKES & KEEPS
Makes almost 750g/1½lb.
Keeps 2 weeks in an airtight container.

METHOD
Cook the ginger in the water for 20 mins until soft. Drain and keep 4 tbs of the cooking water.

Mix the ginger, reserved cooking water and sugar together. Simmer, stirring, for about 20 mins until most of the water has evaporated and the syrup is beginning to crystallize. Then spread the ginger pieces out on a rack to cool.

— *Variation* —

YOU CAN MAKE A SIMILAR MIX USING MARSH MALLOW, ANGELICA, ELECAMPANE, DANDELION AND OTHER ROOTS.

Elderflower Cordial

This delicious cordial is lovely with sparkling water.

INGREDIENTS
- 500g/2½ cups sugar
- 750ml/3 cups boiling water
- 20 heads fresh elderflowers, de-insected as for Elderflower Fritters (p.145)
- 4 lemons, the zest grated and the fruit sliced
- 25g/1oz citric acid powder (a preservative) (optional)

MAKES & KEEPS
Makes approx. 1 litre/1 quart.
Keeps in fridge once opened, use within 3 months.

METHOD
Make a syrup with the sugar and water in a large pan (pp.21–22). Add the elderflowers, lemon zest and pieces and the citric acid, if using, and stir.

Leave to steep with the lid on for 2 days in a cool place, then strain through muslin and bottle.

Use as you would any cordial. Or pour neat over ice cream for a delicious treat.

HERBAL VINEGARS

In herbal vinegars the healing and nutritional properties of vinegar are united with the aromatic and health-protective effects of mineral-rich green herbs. They can be taken as medicines or used in a variety of ways with food: poured over beans or grains, in salad dressings or to season stir-fries and soups.

The following herbal vinegars are made in the same way, with the herbs being left to infuse in the vinegar for several weeks (p.19).

Quantities are provided below as a guide, but often the amount you use will depend upon how much of a particular herb you can find, grow or pick – and on the size of jar you are trying to fill.

For internal use, always make with Apple Cider Vinegar (p.165); for external use (hair and skin washes) or cleaning products, you can use white vinegar if you prefer. For use in laundry rinses make with 1–2 tsp per 250ml/1 cup white vinegar.

If adding to food, try the vinegars in combination with cold-pressed olive oil to make a healthy salad dressing. As a medicine, take 5–10ml/1–2 tsp with a little water, three times a day.

Vinegars will keep for at least 2 years in the fridge.

Ramsons Vinegar

Courtesy of Rachel Corby

This delicious garlicky addition to salad dressings and rice is antioxidant and antiseptic, so also makes for a powerful immune boost.

INGREDIENTS
- 60g/1 cup wild garlic leaves, finely chopped
- 360ml/1½ cups Apple Cider Vinegar (p.165)

MAKES
Makes 360ml/1½ cups.

METHOD
See introduction and key techniques section (left and p.19).

Goldenrod Vinegar

Courtesy of Karen Stephenson

Delicious with pasta and cabbage, this vinegar will improve your mineral balance, help prevent kidney stones, eliminate flatulence and improve immune functioning.

INGREDIENTS
- 30g/1 cup fresh goldenrod leaves and flowers
- 500ml/2 cups Apple Cider Vinegar (p.165)

MAKES
Makes 450ml/almost 2 cups.

METHOD
See introduction and key techniques section (left and p.19).

Cleavers Vinegar

Courtesy of Sensory Solutions

Helps to support the lymphatic system to clear toxins and to cool 'hot' skin conditions such as dermatitis or eczema. It is also used as a diuretic to help with oedema, and to support cancer treatments. Try with wild salad or greens, or as a drink.

INGREDIENTS
- **30g/1 cup fresh cleavers herb**
- **500ml/2 cups Apple Cider Vinegar (p.165)**

MAKES
Makes 450ml/just under 2 cups.

METHOD
See introduction and key techniques section (p.163 and p.19).

Balsamic Vinegar

Courtesy of Karen Stephenson

INGREDIENTS
- **30g/1 cup white pine needles**
- **500ml/2 cups Apple Cider Vinegar (p.165)**

MAKES
Makes 450ml/just under 2 cups.

METHOD
See introduction and key techniques section (p.163 and p.19). Leave the vinegar to infuse for 6 weeks.

Lemon Balm Vinegar

Courtesy of Sensory Solutions

Lemon balm vinegar tastes delicious and goes well with any savoury dish or salad. Lemon balm has been known as 'heart's delight' because of its use to dispel melancholy.

INGREDIENTS
- **30g/1 cup fresh lemon balm flowering tops**
- **500ml/2 cups Apple Cider Vinegar (p.165)**

MAKES
Makes 450ml/just under 2 cups.

METHOD
See introduction and key techniques section (p.163 and p.19).

Oregano Vinegar

Courtesy of Sensory Solutions

Perfect for an Italian-style salad dressing, you can also use it diluted as a gargle for inflamed tonsils or for a head cold. Oregano vinegar is perfect to rebalance gut flora.

INGREDIENTS
- **30g/1 cup fresh oregano flowering tops**
- **500ml/2 cups Apple Cider Vinegar (p.165)**

MAKES
Makes 450ml/just under 2 cups.

METHOD
See introduction and key techniques section (p.163 and p.19).

Rose Vinegar

Makes a lovely pink vinegar with a subtle rose aroma. Good in salad dressings and very useful for the skin and hair. Take as medicine as a liver tonic and an uplifting herb for grieving.

INGREDIENTS
- 30g/1 cup fresh fragrant rose buds or petals
- 500ml/2 cups Apple Cider Vinegar (p.165)

MAKES
Makes 450ml/just under 2 cups.

METHOD
See introduction and key techniques section (p.163 and p.19).

Fire Cider

Courtesy of Karen Stephenson

This spicy hot vinegar goes well with tomato juice or as a straight shot to fight off colds. You can also use it externally as a muscle rub.

INGREDIENTS
- 300ml/1¼ cups Apple Cider Vinegar (p.165)
- 1 fresh horseradish root, grated (making approx. 100g/1 cup)
- 5 garlic cloves, chopped
- 1–2 onions, chopped
- 7.5cm–10cm/3in–4in piece fresh root ginger, grated
- 1 tsp fresh grated cayenne pepper (or ½ tsp dried powdered cayenne if you can't get fresh)

MAKES
Makes 1 litre/1 quart.

METHOD
See introduction and key techniques section for method (p.163 and p.19), steeping for 8 weeks.

Apple Cider Vinegar

Vinegar is made by using a 'mother' — a culture of bacteria which forms during the fermentation process. This mother feeds off the sugars in the fruit, converting them to vinegar.

INGREDIENTS
- 5 apples, quartered
- water – enough to cover

MAKES & KEEPS
Makes a variable amount.
Each batch keeps for 2 years or more.

METHOD
Leave the apples to brown in the air, then place them in a large pot – the pot should be large enough so that they don't come up to the very top – and cover them with water.

Cover the pot with a thin cloth and leave in a warm, dark place. Check it every day, stirring to aerate the mixture and skimming off any froth that comes to the top. After a few days it will start developing a thicker layer on top – this is the vinegar mother beginning to grow. Stop stirring at this point. The liquid will become clearer as the vinegar flavour develops.

After a month, start tasting the mixture by carefully taking a little liquid out with a clean spoon. When you like the tartness, strain the liquid through muslin and bottle it for use. It is normal for a sediment to form in the standing bottles.

Be aware, the first time you brew this it will take a couple of months to get the taste right; however, subsequent batches will be quicker. Once you have your vinegar mother established, you can simply add more water and apple scraps to the jar and leave to ferment.

To clean the jar, carefully remove the mother before lightly rinsing the jar with water. Do not use soap.

Vinegar mothers have been known to last for generations.

Lemon Barley Water

A thirst-quenching drink that is also soothing for the kidneys and bladder. Drink it regularly if you are prone to cystitis.

INGREDIENTS
- 100g/4oz pearl barley
- 1 lemon, zest and juice
- 500ml/2 cups boiling water
- 2–3 tbs honey or sugar

MAKES & KEEPS
Makes 500ml/2 cups.
Drink in 1–2 days. Keep in the fridge.

METHOD
Rinse the barley, then cover it and the lemon zest with boiling water. Simmer for 10 mins, replacing the lost water. Strain the water off and set the barley aside (it is delicious to eat).

Add the lemon juice and honey or sugar to taste.

Easy Cherry Syrup

Delicious on pancakes

INGREDIENTS
- 500ml/2 cups pure cherry juice (a carton is fine)
- 400g/2 cups white sugar

MAKES & KEEPS
Makes approx. 750ml/26fl.oz.
Keeps 3 months in the fridge.

METHOD
Boil the ingredients for 15 mins to make a thickish syrup (pp.21–22).

Chai Tea with Redbush

Adapted from a recipe in **Kitchen of Love** *(2013).*

A delicious, caffeine-free chai.

INGREDIENTS
- 250ml/1 cup water
- 2 redbush tea bags
- 3 cloves
- 1 star anise
- 1 cinnamon stick
- ½ tsp dried ground cinnamon
- ¼ tsp ground black pepper
- 375ml/1½ cups milk or dairy alternative
- sweetener, to taste

SERVES & KEEPS
Serves 2.
Drink immediately.

METHOD
Bring the water, tea bags and spices to the boil. Add the milk and sweetener and simmer for 5–10 mins. Strain and serve.

Saffron & Rose Tea

A lovely tea, rich in antioxidants.

INGREDIENTS
- few strands dried saffron
- 1 dried rosebud
- 1 mug boiling water

MAKES & KEEPS
Makes 1 mug.
Drink immediately.

METHOD
Infuse (p.15) for 5–10 mins. Strain and serve.

Rosemary & Lovage Lemonade

INGREDIENTS
- 1 litre/1 quart water
- 85g/¼ cup honey
- zest from 1 lemon
- juice of 3 lemons
- 3 sprigs fresh rosemary, stripped
- 3 sprigs fresh lovage, chopped
- borage, primrose or nasturtium flowers, to garnish

MAKES & KEEPS
Makes 1 litre/1 quart.
Keeps in the fridge up to 3 days.

METHOD
Boil the water and dissolve the honey in it. Add the zest and leave to cool.

Add the lemon juice and herbs and mix well.

Chill for 2 hours, then serve, garnished with the flowers.

Primrose & Violet Lemonade

INGREDIENTS
- 1 litre/1 quart water
- 85g/¼ cup honey
- zest from 1 lemon
- juice of 3 lemons
- 1 handful of fresh primrose flowers
- ½ handful of fresh violet leaves and flowers
- primrose flowers, to garnish

MAKES & KEEPS
Makes 1 litre/1 quart.
Keeps in the fridge up to 3 days.

METHOD
Make in the same way as Rosemary & Lovage Lemonade (left), but replacing the herbs with the flowers.

Dandelion & Burdock

INGREDIENTS

For the plant 'mother':
- approx. 15cm/6in fresh dandelion root, grated
- approx. 15cm/6in fresh burdock root, grated
- ½ star anise

For the pop:
- 5 litres/1 gallon boiling water
- 340–500g/1½–2½ cups white sugar
- 50g/2oz burdock root, fresh or dry
- 50g/2oz dandelion root, fresh or dry
- juice of 1 lemon or lime

MAKES & KEEPS
Makes 5 litres/1 gallon.
Keeps at least 2–3 months.

METHOD
To make the plant 'mother', make as for Ginger Pop (right), using fresh grated dandelion and burdock roots instead of ginger, and adding ½ star anise to the starter (this gives the drink its hint of aniseed flavour).

Add about 1 tbs of each root every day or two to your starter mix. Usually it's ready to use in about a week.

To make the pop, first decoct each of the roots together with 1 litre/1 quart water for 30 mins (p.15). Add another 3½ litres/¾ gallon boiling water and the sugar (add more if you want it sweeter). Dissolve, add lemon (or lime) juice and leave to cool. Add your strained starter when it has cooled to 26°C/80°F and proceed as for Ginger Pop (right).

Ginger Pop

Making ginger pop is rather like making a home-brewed vinegar. The first time you make it, it takes longer to get the ginger beer 'mother' started, but later batches are quicker.

INGREDIENTS
For the ginger 'mother':
- 250ml/1 cup water
- 7–10 tbs fresh grated root ginger
- white sugar (variable amount)
- 1 tsp baker's yeast

For the pop:
- 340g/1½ cups white sugar
- 15cm/6in piece fresh root ginger, grated (less for a weaker taste)
- 5 litres/1 gallon boiling water
- juice of 1 lemon

YOU WILL NEED
- COOKING THERMOMETER

MAKES & KEEPS
Makes 5 litres/1 gallon.
Keeps at least 2–3 months.

METHOD
To make the ginger beer plant, mix the water with 1 tbs each of ginger and sugar in a jam jar. Sprinkle in the yeast and cover with a cloth or lid. Keep it in a warm place (where you can see it: try also talking to it and inviting it to ferment). Add a little more sugar and ginger every day until it starts bubbling. After about 7–10 days it will be ready.

When you are ready to make the pop, strain the liquid off to use. The 'gunk' left in your sieve or strainer is the ginger beer plant. Feed it with water, sugar and ginger to keep it alive. After a few goes, you can divide it and start one off for a friend.

In a large pan, add the sugar and ginger to the water and simmer for 20 mins. Leave to cool to 26°C/80°F, then add the lemon juice and the liquid you strained off from the plant. Bottle it immediately, leaving at least 7.5cm/3in at the top. Wait a couple of hours before you cork them (sometimes they explode, so choose a cork that can easily pop out).

The pop will be ready to drink in 7–10 days; it will have almost no alcohol content, but will be nice and fizzy.

— *Variation* —

LEAVE TO FERMENT FOR 2–3
DAYS LONGER FOR A STRONGER
ALCOHOLIC BEER.

Yarrow Beer

Adapted from Stephen Buhner's recipe

INGREDIENTS
- 2.2kg/5lb malted barley
- 27 litres/6 gallons water
- 75g/3oz recently dried yarrow (or double the amount fresh)
- 7–14g/¼–½oz brewer's yeast

YOU WILL NEED:
- COOKING THERMOMETER
- FERMENTING VESSEL

MAKES & KEEPS
Makes 25 litres/5 gallons.
Keeps 6–12 months.

METHOD
Preheat the oven to 65°C/150°F/Gas Mark ¼.

'Mash' the barley by roughly crushing it and covering with 5 litres/1 gallon hot water, then place it in the oven for 90 mins.

Next, strain the mixture, keeping the liquid, and 'sparge' the mash – i.e., heat the remaining 25 litres/5 gallons of water and slowly let it drain through the barley mash. Collect all of it and mix with the first liquid.

Add half of the yarrow and bring to the boil. Leave to cool, then pour into a fermenting vessel with the yeast. Put the other half of the yarrow in a muslin bag and hang it in the fermenter. Allow it to ferment until it is finished (normally about 5–7 days), then bottle and cap – at this stage the alcohol content will be negligible. Allow it to ferment in the bottles. After 2 weeks it will be ready to drink.

— *Variation* —

YOU CAN ALSO MAKE THIS AS FOR GINGER POP (P.169) AND DANDELION & BURDOCK (P.168) – THE LONGER YOU LEAVE IT FERMENTING (FROM 7–21 DAYS), THE STRONGER IT GETS.

Nettle Beer

Courtesy of Susun Weed

A delightful drink which can be taken as a medicine for joint pain.

INGREDIENTS
- 500g/2½ cups raw sugar
- juice and peel of 2 lemons
- 30g/1oz cream of tartar
- 1kg/8 pints fresh chopped nettles
- 5 litres/1 gallon water
- 30g/1oz fresh yeast

MAKES & KEEPS
Makes 5 litres/1 gallon.
Keeps at least 2–3 months.

METHOD
Place the sugar, lemon peel (no pith), lemon juice and cream of tartar in a large casserole dish with a lid. Cook the nettles in the water for 15 mins. Strain into the casserole and stir well. When this cools to blood temperature, dissolve the yeast in a little water and add to your casserole.

Cover with several folds of cloth and leave it to brew for 3 days. Strain out the sediment and bottle. It will be ready to drink in 8 days.

Elderflower Champagne

INGREDIENTS
- 1 lemon
- 350g/1¾ cups sugar
- 1 tbs wine vinegar
- 12 fresh elderflower heads
- 4½ litres/1 gallon boiling water
- 2¼ litres/2 quarts cold water

MAKES & KEEPS
Makes 2 litres/2 quarts.
Keeps up to 12 months.

METHOD
In a scrupulously clean large bowl, add the juice and zest of ½ lemon, and add the other half, sliced. Add the sugar, vinegar and flowers. Bruise with a potato masher. Add the boiling water and stir for several minutes. Leave for 1–2 hours, then add the cold water, cover with cloth and leave for 2–4 days. Strain through muslin and bottle it with corks.

Store for 7–10 days before drinking.

Dandelion Champagne

INGREDIENTS
- 1 litre/1 quart fresh dandelion flowers, stalks removed, fully opened
- 4½ litres/1 gallon boiling water
- 350g/1¾ cups sugar
- juice of 2 lemons
- 1 tbs wine vinegar
- 2¼ litres/2 quarts cold water

MAKES & KEEPS
Makes 6½ litres/1½ gallons.
Keeps 6–12 months.

METHOD
Cover the flowers with the boiling water. Mix in the sugar and leave for 12 hours. Strain and add the lemon juice, vinegar and cold water.

Bottle, cork and leave to brew (10 days for a non-alcoholic fizz and 3–4 weeks for a mildly alcoholic version).

Dandelion Coffee

Courtesy of Annie Powell

A delicious and healthy alternative to coffee.

INGREDIENTS

Dandelion roots, as many 5cm/2in-long roots as you can find, scrubbed, chopped and dried for 24 hours by a radiator

Place the roots in a single layer on a baking tray in the oven at the lowest temperature. Cook very slowly for 2–5 hours (depending upon the temperature of your oven) until the roots look charred, dark brown/black and withered. Leave to cool thoroughly for 1–2 hours. Store in jars until use.

KEEPS
Roasted roots will keep up to a year in an airtight container.
Once brewed, drink immediately.

METHOD
Put a pan of water on to heat. Add some dried dandelion root (about 3 x 5cm/2in-long pieces should be enough for a cup). Bring to the boil and simmer for 10–15 mins. By this time the water will be dark brown. Strain into cups and drink, adding milk and sugar to taste, if required.

RECREATIONAL TINCTURES

'Recreational' tinctures are tinctures that have been sweetened with sugar or honey to make a tasty alcoholic drink. They are all made as for ordinary tinctures, by mixing the ingredients and leaving them to steep for some weeks, then straining and bottling (pp.18–19).

The following recipes will make 700ml/ almost 2 cups and keep for years – though they are so nice they are unlikely to be given the chance! You can drink them neat in small glasses, mixed with sparkling water to make a refreshing drink or made into a hot punch, mixed with boiling water.

Pear & Nutmeg Brandy

This is one of my most popular drinks, as it is absolutely gorgeous.

INGREDIENTS
- 4–5 pears, cut up
- 2 whole nutmegs, freshly grated
- 750ml/3 cups brandy (the best you can afford)
- 2 tbs honey

METHOD
See introduction and key techniques section (left and pp.18–19).

Aphrodisiac Brandy

INGREDIENTS
- 100g/4oz dried ground ginseng root
- 100g/4oz dried ground rhodiola rosea powder
- 4 cinnamon sticks, broken up
- 4 whole vanilla pods
- 2–6 whole chillies (depends on taste as they will be hot!)
- 750ml/3 cups brandy
- 2 tbs honey

METHOD
See introduction and key techniques section (left and pp.18–19).

FOOD & DRINK

Sloe Vodka

Courtesy of Lynn Amanda Brown

A variation on the traditional sloe gin.

INGREDIENTS
- 450g/about 3 cups fresh sloes
- 750ml/3 cups vodka
- 350g/1¾ cups sugar

METHOD
See introduction and key techniques section (left and pp.18–19).

Plum Mead

- 4 generous handfuls of fresh sweet plums
- 750ml/3 cups mead (honey wine)
- 1–2 tbs muscovado sugar
- 1–2 tsp each ground cinnamon and nutmeg (optional)

METHOD
See introduction and key techniques section (left and pp.18–19).

Mabon Welcome Cup (Blackberry & Blackcurrant Brandy)

A Celtic tradition, the welcome cup was a special drink, often strong liqueur (with strong magic in it), offered to all at the start of a ceremony.

INGREDIENTS
- 1–2 large handfuls of fresh blackberries
- 1–2 large handfuls of fresh blackcurrants
- 750ml/3 cups brandy
- 1 tbs honey

METHOD
See introduction and key techniques section (left and pp.18–19).

Very Berry Mead

A delicious and enjoyable drink, packed with vitamin C.

INGREDIENTS
1 generous handful of each of these fresh fruits:
- raspberries
- rowan berries
- hawthorn berries
- blackberries
- bilberries (or blueberries)

- 750ml/3 cups mead (honey wine)
- 1 tbs soft brown sugar, dissolved in 2 tbs hot water

METHOD
See introduction and key techniques section (left and pp.18–19).

Horseradish Vodka

Good with tomato juice or try it straight as a shot with lime juice and salt to wake you up. It is also a medicine which helps to stimulate the immune system and the circulation.

INGREDIENTS
- 100g/1 cup fresh grated horseradish
- 750ml/3 cups vodka

METHOD
See introduction and key techniques section (p.172 and pp.18–19).

If taking medicinally, take 1–2 tsp 1–2 times day.

Gorse Liqueur

Gorse is uplifting and cheering.

INGREDIENTS
- 4 handfuls of fresh gorse flowers
- 1–2 tbs honey
- 750ml/3 cups half and half vodka and mead mixed

METHOD
See introduction and key techniques section (p.172 and pp.18–19).

Drink sparingly – beware, it is very strong.

Medicinal Port Brandy

Courtesy of ChaNan Bonser

This is very delicious and of course highly medicinal … you can use it for coughs, bronchial issues, at the first sign of a cold or flu, you can have little sips, mix with honey to taste and also serve warm if you like.

INGREDIENTS
- 50g/2 cups freshly picked elderberries
- 500ml/2 cups port wine
- 500ml/2 cups brandy
- 2 cinnamon sticks
- 1 tsp dried ginger (or about 2.5cm/1in of fresh root ginger)
- 6 cardamom pods
- 8 black peppercorns
- 8 cloves

MAKES & KEEPS
Makes just under 1 litre/1 quart.
Keeps at least 2–3 years.

METHOD
See introduction and key techniques section (p.172 and pp.18–19).

— *Tip* —

ADJUST THE SPICES TO YOUR TASTE, ADDING MORE OR LESS AS YOU LIKE.

Swiss Gentian Aperitif Wine

Courtesy of Christine Herren-Valette

This fortified wine is good as both an aperitif (a pre-dinner drink) and a digestive (taken after the meal). Gentian is an excellent liver stimulant that aids digestion. Yellow gentian is a digestive, reduces fever and is a general tonic.

INGREDIENTS
- 40g/¾ cup fresh root of yellow gentian, roughly chopped
- 250ml/1 cup apple schnapps (60% proof)
- 2.5 litres/½ gallon white wine
- zest of 1 lemon
- zest of 2 oranges
- 125ml/½ cup water
- 600g/3 cups sugar

MAKES & KEEPS
Makes 3 litres/¾ gallon.
Keeps 1 year.

METHOD
Mix the chopped gentian root and apple schnapps. Cover and leave to macerate for 48 hours. Then add the white wine and the lemon and orange zest and re-cover.

Leave for 10 days in a dark place, stirring a little every 2 days.

After 10 days strain and press through muslin. Make a syrup (pp.21–22) by boiling the water and sugar together for 1 min.

Mix the syrup and gentian wine and bottle.

— *Tip* —

THERE IS OFTEN A DEPOSIT ON THE SURFACE OF THE GENTIAN WINE, BUT DO NOT THROW AWAY. JUST STIR OR SHAKE THE BOTTLE TO REMIX AS IT IS DELICIOUS.

Angelica Archangel After-dinner Liqueur

Courtesy of Christine Herren

INGREDIENTS
- 300g/2 cups fresh stalks angelica, cut to 1cm/½in in length (wash and dry with tea towel after picking)
- 3 cloves
- 2 litres/½ gallon apple spirit (40% proof)
- 400ml/1¾ cups water
- 430g/2 cups + 2 tbs sugar

MAKES & KEEPS
Makes 2.5 litres/½ gallon.
Keeps 5 years.

METHOD
Put the chopped angelica stalks, cloves and apple spirit in a large glass jar. Leave covered in a dark place for 2 months. Strain and press.

Make a syrup (pp.21–22) by boiling the water and sugar together for 1 min.

Mix this with the angelica liqueur and then pour into bottles.

THE RECIPES

HOMEMADE WINE

Wine can be made from anything edible. Whatever sort of wine you choose to make, the flowers/leaves/fruit should be at their prime and picked on a dry, preferably sunny day and placed in plastic measuring jugs. The following simple method, kindly given by Annie Powell, uses no chemicals or additives, other than wine yeast, and can be used for all the wine recipes here.

YOU WILL NEED

- LARGE PLASTIC BUCKET OR CERAMIC CASSEROLE DISH
- DEMIJOHN, BUNG AND AIRLOCK (MUST BE THOROUGHLY CLEAN: SIMMER THE AIRLOCK AND BUNG FOR 5 MINS, RINSE AND PUT CLEAN WATER IN THE AIRLOCK)
- PLASTIC FUNNEL
- COTTON MUSLIN (BIG ENOUGH TO COVER MOUTH OF BUCKET/CASSEROLE DISH, WITH 7.5CM/3IN OVERLAP ALL ROUND
- STRING (ENOUGH TO GO ROUND MOUTH OF BUCKET/CASSEROLE DISH WITH 15CM/6IN TO SPARE)
- BOTTLE BRUSH
- BLACK BIN BAG
- SYPHON TUBE

MAKES & KEEPS
Each recipe makes 4½ litres/1 gallon, and can keep for years.

METHOD
Place the flowers or leaves in the bucket/casserole dish.

Boil half of the water and pour it over them. Add the lemon juice and cover the bucket with muslin tied with string. Leave for 3 days, shaking or stirring several times a day.

Boil the remaining water with the sugar. Add to the infused flowers or leaves and stir. Leave to cool until lukewarm/hand-hot, then add the yeast. Leave for 1 hour.

Stir and strain the mixture through the cotton muslin into the demijohn using a funnel (this is a two-person job) and fit the bung and airlock. Place the demijohn in a black bin (which keeps it warm and dark). Leave it in a warm place.

Within 24 hours (sometimes within minutes!) it should start 'blipping' (fermenting). If it hasn't within 24 hours, give it a shake. If nothing happens after another hour or 2, add another 1 tsp yeast. Different wines ferment at different rates; when it has stopped 'blipping' for a couple of weeks syphon off into a clean demijohn or bottles. Leave for at least 3 months before drinking.

Gorse Wine

Courtesy of Annie Powell

To pick gorse flowers, grasp them between your thumb and index finger and pull. Only the yellow flowers are used, none of the green, and watch out for the spikes.

INGREDIENTS
- 4½ litres/1 gallon water
- 1 litre/2 pints fresh gorse flowers
- juice of 2 lemons
- 900g/4 cups granulated sugar
- 1 rounded tsp wine yeast

Walnut Leaf Wine

Courtesy of Annie Powell

INGREDIENTS
- 4½ litres/1 gallon water
- 3 good sprigs of fresh walnut leaves, crushed gently by hand
- juice of 2 lemons
- 900g/4 cups granulated sugar
- 1 rounded tsp wine yeast

Elderflower Wine

A favourite wine, perfect to make hayfever and cough medicine tinctures from.

INGREDIENTS
- 4½ litres/1 gallon water
- 2 litres/2 quarts elderflowers
- juice of 2 lemons
- 900g/4 cups granulated sugar
- 1 rounded tsp wine yeast

Oak Leaf Wine

Makes a good medium-dry white.

INGREDIENTS
- 4½ litres/1 gallon water
- 5 litres/9 quarts fresh oak leaves
- juice of 2 lemons
- 900g/4 cups granulated sugar
- 1 rounded tsp wine yeast

Ashwagandha Night Cap

Courtesy of Anne McIntyre

Ashwagandha is a wonderful Ayurvedic herb with deeply relaxing and stress-busting properties.

INGREDIENTS
- 1 tsp ashwagandha powder
- 1 mug warm almond milk
- 1 tsp rosewater
- pinch of cardamom powder

MAKES & KEEPS
Makes 1 mug.
Drink fresh.

METHOD
Warm the ingredients together.
Sip before bedtime for a restful sleep.

BEAUTY, BALMS & PERSONAL CARE

You can make your own all-natural beauty and personal care products which rely on the wonderful power of plants – from cleanser to lipstick through body butter, from soap and shampoo to shaving cream and deodorant. These preparations contain pure ingredients which enhance your health and feed and nourish your skin. Treat yourself and care for the environment at the same time.

Cleopatra's Cleanser

Courtesy of Teri Evans

Great for make-up removal. This is based on a recipe used by Cleopatra – she wouldn't have had grapefruit seed extract, but she would have had asses' milk…

INGREDIENTS
- 3 tbs + 1 tsp olive oil
- 8 tsp aloe vera gel
- 2 tbs rosewater
- 4 drops rose essential oil
- 2 drops grapefruit seed extract

MAKES & KEEPS
Makes 120ml/½ cup.
Keeps 6 months.

METHOD
Whisk the olive oil into the aloe vera. Continue whisking while you gradually add the rosewater. Add the rose essential oil and grapefruit seed extract and whisk well. Pour or spoon into a jar.

Massage into your face and neck twice daily. Either wash off with a flannel (then tone and moisturize) or remove with cotton wool (then it will act as a moisturizer too).

Mint Chocolate Face Pack

Courtesy of Teri Evans

Deeply cleansing, like all face masks, and really good fun. It smells divine – almost good enough to eat!

INGREDIENTS
- 1½ tbs raw cocoa powder
- 1 tbs white kaolin powder
- 10g/½ cup dried peppermint leaves
- 40–60ml/up to ¼ cup coconut oil

MAKES & KEEPS
Makes almost 250ml/1 cup.
Keeps up to 6 months in a jar.

METHOD
Mix the dry ingredients together. Gradually add the oil until you have a thick paste.

Apply to cleansed skin and then leave on for 15–20 mins. Wash off well and moisturize.

— Variation —
YOU CAN SUBSTITUTE COCONUT MILK FOR THE COCONUT OIL AND REPLACE DRIED HERBS WITH THE SAME QUANTITY OF FRESH IF YOU WILL BE USING IT IMMEDIATELY.

Soothing Face Mask

Courtesy of Teri Evans

Suitable for all skin types, especially dry and irritated. These quantities will give you 2 applications — or share with a friend.

INGREDIENTS
- 3 tbs white clay/ kaolin powder
- 1½ tbs milk powder

Essential oils:
- 1 drop frankincense
- 1 drop chamomile
- 1 tsp lavender water (possibly more)

MAKES & KEEPS
Makes 2 masks.
Use immediately.

METHOD
Mix the dry ingredients together. Add the essential oils and lavender water and stir well. Leave for a few minutes, and then if necessary add more lavender water until you have a consistency that is easy to spread.

Use as described for Mint Chocolate Face Pack (opposite).

Nourishing & Cleansing Face Mask

Courtesy of ChaNan Bonser

A super-simple recipe, ready in an instant. Suitable for all skin types.

INGREDIENTS
- splash of rosewater
- splash of witch hazel
- 1½ tsp gram (chickpea) flour

MAKES & KEEPS
Makes 1 mask.
Use immediately.

METHOD
Mix the rosewater and witch hazel with the gram (chickpea) flour to form a paste.

Use as described for Mint Chocolate Face Pack (opposite).

Yarrow Soothing Skin Wash

Courtesy of Maida Silverman

Yarrow makes an excellent astringent skin wash, especially suitable for oily skin.

INGREDIENTS
- **500ml/2 cups boiling water**
- **20g/½ cup dried yarrow flowering tops, crumbled**

MAKES & KEEPS
Makes just under 500ml/2 cups.
Keeps in the fridge for 4–5 days.

METHOD
Pour the water over the yarrow flowers, leave to cool for 30–60 mins and then strain.

Pat it on the skin frequently to soothe irritation.

Lavender Toner

Courtesy of Teri Evans

This is a super-easy toner suitable for all skin types, especially blemished.

INGREDIENTS
- 4 tbs vodka
- 4 tbs lavender water (or rose, orange-flower or other floral water as preferred)
- drizzle of vegetable glycerine
- 9 drops lavender essential oil

MAKES & KEEPS
Makes 120ml/½ cup.
Keeps 1 year.

METHOD
Pour all the ingredients into a bottle and shake well to mix.

Shake before use. Use daily, applying with cotton wool after cleansing. Avoid eye area.

Gentle Rose Toner for Mature Skin

INGREDIENTS
- 100ml/just under ½ cup rosewater
- 1 tbs Rose Vinegar (p.165)
- 1 tsp glycerine

Essential oils:
- 6 drops rose
- 6 drops rose geranium

MAKES & KEEPS
Makes 120ml/½ cup.
Keeps 6 months.

METHOD
Pour all the ingredients into a bottle and shake well to mix.

Use as for Lavender Toner (above).

Wintertime Facial Toner

Courtesy of Jenny Pao

A facial toning elixir for all skin types. It soothes irritated skin, tightens pores and keeps acne at bay.

INGREDIENTS
- 375ml/1½ cups water
- 1 peppermint tea bag
- 1 rooibos tea bag
- 1 chamomile tea bag

Essential oils:
- 1 drop rosemary
- 4 drops lavender

MAKES & KEEPS
Makes 375ml/1½ cups.
Keeps 2 weeks in the fridge.

METHOD
Bring the water to the boil, then leave to cool for 3 mins. Pour the water over the tea bags in a pot and leave to stand for 5 mins.

Cool completely before removing the tea bags. Add the oils and pour into a glass bottle.

Shake bottle before use. Apply toner daily to clean skin prior to moisturizing.

BEAUTY, BALMS & PERSONAL CARE

Medicinal Lavender Skin Tonic

Courtesy of Teri Evans

Suitable for all skins, the apple cider vinegar makes it especially good for problem skins. The smell does not linger once applied.

INGREDIENTS
- **2 handfuls of lavender flowers**
- **225ml/just under 1 cup Apple Cider Vinegar (p.165)**
- **700ml/just under 3 cups rosewater or Lavender Water (p.134)**

MAKES & KEEPS
Makes 900ml/almost 3¾ cups.
Keeps at least 1 year.

METHOD
Put the lavender flowers in the bottom of a large jar. Pour in the vinegar and rosewater and shake to ensure there are no air bubbles. Let it infuse for 1–2 weeks, shaking the jar occasionally. Strain through muslin.

Shake before use. Apply daily after cleansing.

— *Variation* —

FOR A POWERFUL LOTION TO TREAT ACNE AND INTERTRIGO (A FUNGAL-TYPE INFECTION THAT CAUSES SORENESS IN SKIN FOLDS), ADD THESE ESSENTIAL OILS TO THE ABOVE LOTION:
- 100 drops/1 tsp tea tree
- 100 drops/1 tsp lavender
- 50 drops/½ tsp thyme

APPLY THE LOTION 2–3 TIMES DAILY TO SORE AREAS.

Simple Rose Face Cream

Courtesy of Lynn Rawlinson

This is the simplest cream you can make.

INGREDIENTS
Oil fraction:
- 100g/½ cup coconut oil
- 25ml/5 tsp avocado oil
- 1 tbs honey

Water fraction:
- 5 tsp rosewater

At the end:
- 10–15 drops rose (or rose geranium) essential oil (optional)

MAKES & KEEPS
Makes 175ml/¾ cup.
Keeps 6–12 months.

METHOD
Melt the coconut and avocado oils and the honey in a bain-marie, then gently warm the rosewater in a separate bowl in the bain-marie. Remove from the heat, and start to whisk the oil and honey mixture. As you do so, add a drop of rosewater.

Keep whisking and adding a little rosewater until you have used all of it, then whisk until the mixture starts to solidify. When it is semi-solid, add the essential oils and whisk until well blended. Store in sterilized jars.

Rosy Lotion

Courtesy of Teri Evans

A nice, light lotion suitable as a face moisturizer for all skin types, including oily skin.

It is also good as a non-greasy hand-nourisher for people who find hand creams too rich.

INGREDIENTS
- 100ml/just under ½ cup rosewater
- 100ml/just under ½ cup glycerine
- 50 drops/½ tsp rose geranium essential oil

MAKES & KEEPS
Makes 200ml/1¾ cups.
Keeps 6 months.

METHOD
Whisk all the ingredients in a jug for a couple of minutes until they are blended. Then pour into a bottle.

Shake before use. Massage a small amount into your hands until absorbed.

Anti-ageing Day Cream

Courtesy of Teri Evans

This has all the ingredients of a top quality, super-expensive skin cream from a laboratory. Carrot oil contains vitamin A, which helps to improve the elasticity of collagen and plump up your skin. Vitamin C is a free-radical scavenger — antioxidants help to slow down the effects of ageing, basically reducing damage from UV rays. Rose helps to heal broken capillaries and reduces wrinkles, and glycerine helps to hold moisture in your skin.

Creams can be tricky to make, so before starting read the guidance on pp. 20–21.

INGREDIENTS
Oil fraction:
- 2.5g/½ tsp beeswax
- 5g/1 tsp emulsifying wax
- 28g/2 tbs mango or shea butter
- 15ml/1 tbs carrot oil
- 15ml/1 tbs evening primrose oil
- 2.5g/½ tsp vitamin C powder
- 5ml/½ tsp glycerine

Water fraction:
- 85ml/5 tbs rosewater

Extras:
- 10 drops rose essential oil

MAKES & KEEPS
Makes about 120g/½ cup.
Keeps at least 2–3 months.

METHOD
Gently heat the waxes, mango or shea butter and carrot and evening primrose oils together in a bain-marie. When the waxes have melted, add the vitamin C powder and glycerine, and whisk well to mix.

Warm the rosewater to the same temperature. Whisk the rosewater into the oil fraction mix, adding the rose essential oil when the cream is cool.

Apply a small amount each morning to the face and neck.

Intensive Eye Serum

Courtesy of Monika Ghent

Oils can also be blended for different purposes. Use this eye serum for around the eye to treat dark circles or ageing skin.

INGREDIENTS
- oil from 5 vitamin E capsules (400 IU)
- 7ml/1½ tsp camellia seed oil
- 7ml/1½ tsp rosehip seed oil
- 10ml/2 tsp argan oil

Essential oils:
- 10 drops carrot seed
- 10 drops lemon
- 5 drops fennel
- 5 drops geranium
- 5 drops patchouli
- 5 drops rosemary
- 20 drops lavender

MAKES & KEEPS
Makes 25ml/5 tsp.
Keeps at least 6 months.

METHOD
Place all the ingredients in a dropper bottle and shake well.

Apply a few drops twice daily to the skin around the eyes.

Facial Serum for Sun-damaged Skin

Courtesy of Monika Ghent

This serum of blended oils repairs sun damage at the cellular level.

INGREDIENTS
- 7ml/1½ tsp camellia seed oil
- 7ml/1½ tsp argan oil
- 7ml/1½ tsp rosehip seed oil
- 5ml/1 tsp jojoba oil
- oil from 5 vitamin E capsules (400 IU)
- 10 drops of liquid vitamin D

Essential oils:
- 25 drops lavender
- 10 drops lemon
- 10 drops carrot seed
- 10 drops palma rosa
- 5 drops rosemary
- 5 drops patchouli
- 5 drops geranium

MAKES & KEEPS
Makes 30ml/1oz bottle
(best to use pump spray dispenser).
Keeps 6 months in the fridge.

METHOD
Combine all the ingredients in a bottle and shake well.

Apply to the face 1–2 times daily.

Tropical Body Buff

Courtesy of Teri Evans

To exfoliate and nourish the skin.

INGREDIENTS
- 100g/½ cup coconut oil
- 245g/1¼ cups brown or raw sugar

Essential oils:
- 6 drops orange
- 4 drops lemongrass
- 3 drops ylang-ylang

MAKES & KEEPS
Makes 250g/up to 2½ cups.
Keeps 6 months.

METHOD
Warm the coconut oil in a bain-marie until it is just melted. Blend with the sugar well. Add the essential oils, making sure to mix well.

To use, massage a little into damp skin and wash off with warm water.

Caution
Do not use on damaged skin or on acne.

Choca-coco Sugar Body Scrub

Courtesy of Monika Ghent

INGREDIENTS
- 100g/just under ½ cup coconut oil
- 200g/1 cup whole cane sugar
- 60g/¼ cup coconut sugar
- 2 tbs cocoa powder
- 2 tbs jojoba oil
- 1 tsp vanilla extract
- **oil from 5 vitamin E capsules (400 IU)**

MAKES & KEEPS
Makes 3 x 125ml/½ cup-sized jam jars.
Keeps up to 1 year.

METHOD
Gently melt the coconut oil in a bain-marie, then blend with the rest of the ingredients in a mixing bowl before decanting into jars.

Use as for Tropical Body Buff (left).

BEAUTY, BALMS & PERSONAL CARE

Exfoliating Seaweed Scrub

Courtesy of Teri Evans

INGREDIENTS
- 1 tbs fine sea salt
- 1 tbs kelp powder
- 5 tsp vegetable glycerine
- 7 tsp sweet almond oil

Essential oils:
- 5 drops juniper
- 5 drops lemon

MAKES & KEEPS
Makes 100g/just under ½ cup.
Keeps at least 6 months.

METHOD
Mix the sea salt and kelp together. Add the glycerine and half the almond oil and mix well. If the mixture is too stiff, add more oil until it makes a thick, gloopy paste.

Add the essential oils and stir really well. Use as for Tropical Body Buff (opposite).

Note: not suitable for dry skin.

Anti-cellulite Body Scrub

INGREDIENTS
- 1 tbs fine sea salt
- 1 tbs ground coffee
- 5 tsp vegetable glycerine
- 7 tsp sweet almond oil

Essential oils:
- 5 drops juniper
- 5 drops grapefruit

MAKES & KEEPS
Makes 100g/just under ½ cup.
Keeps at least 6 months.

METHOD
Make and use as for Exfoliating Seaweed Scrub (above), adding the coffee in place of the kelp.

— *Tip* —
LEAVE THE SEA SALT OUT OF YOUR SCRUB RECIPES AND USE THEM AS BODY MASKS INSTEAD. SPREAD OVER YOUR BODY, LEAVE ON FOR 20 MINS AND THEN RINSE OFF.

Rosy Bath Bomb

Courtesy of Teri Evans

INGREDIENTS
- 600g/2½ cups bicarbonate of soda
- 2 tsp rosehip oil
- 2 tsp dry rose petals
- 300g/¾ cup citric acid

Essential oils:
- 30 drops rose geranium
- 30 drops jasmine

- few drops red food colouring
- water in a spray bottle

YOU WILL NEED
- MOULDS FOR CUPCAKE-SIZE BOMBS

MAKES & KEEPS
Makes 12 bombs the size of cupcake cases (fewer if larger).
Keeps up to 1 year in an airtight container. (Note: they can't go off, but the smell slowly disappears as the essential oils evaporate.)

METHOD
Combine all the dry ingredients in a bowl and mix well. Mix the oils together, then add to the powders and mix again.

Add the food colouring to the water, then spray a little amount of water over the mix and blend in quickly and thoroughly. It has enough water added when you can squeeze it together and it only just holds together. Press very firmly into moulds. Leave for up to ½ hour to set, then turn out carefully.

Relaxation Bath Salts

Courtesy of Lucy Harmer

INGREDIENTS
- 1kg/3½ cups sea salt or natural rock salt
- 30g/1oz dried lavender flowers
- 20g/⅔oz dried chamomile flowers

Essential oils:
- 21 drops lavender
- 21 drops chamomile

MAKES & KEEPS
Makes just over 1kg/4½ cups.
Keeps 1 year.

METHOD
Mix together and then keep in a sealed glass jar.

Add a small handful to your bath as required.

Love Spell Bath Salts

Courtesy of Lucy Harmer

I like to use Himalayan salt as it's naturally pink.

INGREDIENTS
- 1kg/3½ cups sea salt or natural rock salt
- 25g/1oz dried damascus rose petals

Essential oils:
- 14 drops damascus rose
- 14 drops geranium
- 14 drops palmarosa

MAKES & KEEPS
Makes 1kg/4½ cups.
Keeps 1 year.

METHOD
Mix all the ingredients together well and then keep in a sealed glass jar.

Add a small handful to your bath as required.

Purification Bath Salts

Courtesy of Lucy Harmer

INGREDIENTS
- 1kg/3½ cups sea salt or natural rock salt
- 50g/2oz dried lavender flowers

Essential oils:
- 20 drops lavender
- 10 drops rosemary
- 10 drops juniper

MAKES & KEEPS
Makes just over 1kg/4½ cups.
Keeps 1 year.

METHOD
Mix all the ingredients together well and then keep in a sealed glass jar.

Add a small handful to your bath as required.

Fruity Body Custard

Courtesy of Teri Evans

This light but deeply nourishing moisturizer is almost good enough to eat.

INGREDIENTS
- 2 tbs + 1 tsp apricot kernel oil
- 1 tbs jojoba oil
- 2 tbs aloe vera gel
- 2 tbs orange-flower water

Essential oils:
- 10 drops sweet orange
- 3 drops pink grapefruit
- 2 drops bergamot

- 2 drops grapefruit seed extract

MAKES & KEEPS
Makes 120ml/½ cup.
Keeps 6 months.

METHOD
Whisk the apricot kernel and jojoba oils into the aloe vera gel. Gradually add the orange-flower water while whisking until the mixture thickens and becomes creamy. Add the essential oils and grapefruit seed extract.

Massage into the skin as required.

[Invigorating Body Butter]

Courtesy of Teri Evans

A rich body moisturizer (richer than Fruity Body Custard, left).

INGREDIENTS
- 2 tbs cocoa butter
- 4 tbs shea butter
- 2 tbs coconut oil
- 4 tbs evening primrose oil

Essential oils:
- 10 drops rosemary
- 10 drops lemon
- 5 drops ginger

MAKES & KEEPS
Makes 250ml/1 cup.
Keeps 6 months.

METHOD
Gently heat the cocoa and shea butters with the coconut oil in a bain-marie until they have melted. Remove from the heat and cool until hand-hot. Add the evening primrose oil and essential oils and whisk well.

The butter won't set at room temperature. For best results, put the bowl in the fridge, removing every 30 mins or so to whisk. When nearly set, whisk well and pour into jars. Replace in the fridge until finally set.

Luxurious Body Butter

INGREDIENTS
- 2 tbs cocoa butter
- 4 tbs shea butter
- 2 tbs coconut oil
- 4 tbs evening primrose oil

Essential oils:
- 10 drops jasmine
- 10 drops sandalwood
- 5 drops rose

MAKES & KEEPS
Makes 250ml/1 cup.
Keeps 6 months.

METHOD
Make as for All-invigorating Body Butter (p.187).

Antiseptic Body Butter

Good for skin prone to spots.

INGREDIENTS
- 2 tbs cocoa butter
- 4 tbs shea butter
- 2 tbs coconut oil
- 4 tbs evening primrose oil

Essential oils:
- 10 drops tea tree
- 10 drops oregano
- 5 drops thyme

MAKES & KEEPS
Makes 250ml/1 cup.
Keeps 6 months.

METHOD
Make as for All-invigorating Body Butter (p.187).

Revive Facial Mist

Courtesy of Monika Ghent

A pick-me-up throughout the day, this also helps to combat dry skin and uplift the spirits in winter.

INGREDIENTS
- 200ml/¾ cup + 3 tbs still mineral water
- 2 tbs rosewater
- 1 tsp glycerine
- 2 tsp witch hazel

Essential oils:
- 6 drops spearmint
- 5 drops rosemary
- 3 drops palmarosa

MAKES & KEEPS
Makes 250ml/1 cup.
Keeps 1–2 months.

METHOD
Measure all the ingredients directly into a spray bottle.

To use, shake well, close your eyes and spray on to your face.

Lavender & Rose Handcream

Courtesy of Teri Evans

Creams can be tricky to make, so before starting read the guidance on pp. 20–21.

INGREDIENTS
Oil fraction:
- 115ml/just under ½ cup coconut oil
- 21g/2½ tbs beeswax
- 15g/1 tbs cocoa butter

Water fraction:
- 75ml/¼ cup + 1 tbs rosewater
- 2.5g/½ tsp borax (see box, p.43)

Essential oils:
- 10 drops rose
- 8 drops geranium
- 5 drops ylang-ylang
- 15 drops lavender

MAKES & KEEPS
Makes 210g/nearly 1 cup.
Keeps 2–3 months.

METHOD
Heat the oil fraction ingredients together in a bain-marie. Then take off the heat and let it cool slightly. Meanwhile, gently heat the water fraction until the borax dissolves.

Whisk the oil mix briskly until the bowl is hand-warm. Gradually add the water fraction ingredients without stopping whisking. Whisk as though your life depended on it! When the mixture looks creamy and white add the essential oils while still whisking. You will notice a point when the cream starts to set: at this point, pour into jars.

Timing is the key with this recipe. If you leave it too late, you will have to scrape the cream into the jars. If you pour too soon, the cream will separate.

Antiseptic Handcream

INGREDIENTS
Oil fraction:
- 115ml/just under ½ cup coconut oil
- 21g/2½ tsp beeswax
- 15g/1 tbs cocoa butter

Water fraction:
- 75ml/¼ cup + 1 tbs lavender water or witch hazel
- 2.5g/½ tsp borax (see box, p.43)

Essential oils:
- 12 drops thyme
- 12 drops tea tree
- 12 drops oregano

MAKES & KEEPS
Makes 210g/nearly 1 cup.
Keeps 2–3 months.

METHOD
Make as for Lavender & Rose Handcream (left).

Nail & Cuticle Booster

Courtesy of Teri Evans

INGREDIENTS
- 10g/⅓oz dried horsetail
- 4 tbs sunflower oil
- 3 drops lemon essential oil

MAKES & KEEPS
Makes about 60ml/¼ cup.
Keeps up to 6 months.

METHOD
Make an infused oil with the horsetail and sunflower oil (p.20). Add the lemon essential oil and bottle.

Massage a little oil into your cuticles at night to stimulate blood flow.

— *Tip* —

FOR A DEEP NAIL-STRENGTHENING TREATMENT, WARM THE OIL GENTLY IN A BAIN-MARIE AND SOAK YOUR NAILS IN IT FOR 20 MINS. YOU CAN RE-USE THE OIL AGAIN AND AGAIN.

Nourishing Nail Oil

Courtesy of Monika Ghent

Use this oil to strengthen and protect dry, brittle nails.

INGREDIENTS
- 2 tsp jojoba oil
- 1 tbs sweet almond oil
- oil from 5 vitamin E capsules (400 IU)

Essential oils:
- 25 drops lavender
- 8 drops rosemary
- 6 drops spearmint
- 4 drops black spruce

MAKES & KEEPS
Makes 25ml/5 tsp.
Keeps around 6 months.

METHOD
Add all the other ingredients to a dropper bottle and shake well.

Apply 2–3 times daily to nails and nail bed.

Foot & Leg Spray

Courtesy of Teri Evans

This helps to treat smelly feet, as well as to soothe and tone aching varicose veins.

INGREDIENTS
- 100ml/just under ½ cup witch hazel
- 1 tsp bicarbonate of soda

Essential oils:
- 10 drops peppermint
- 8 drops rosemary
- 5 drops bergamot

MAKES & KEEPS
Makes 100ml/just under ½ cup.
Keeps 1 year.

METHOD
Gently heat the witch hazel and bicarbonate of soda until the bicarbonate is dissolved. Add the oils and store in a spray bottle.

Shake before use. Spray on your legs and feet 1–2 times daily.

Soothing & Refreshing Foot Bath

Courtesy of Johanna Herzog

This helps to protect against athlete's foot, and to treat aching and sweaty feet.

INGREDIENTS
- 2 handfuls of birch buds or leaves
- 2 handfuls of leaves and bark of ivy
- 1 litre/1 quart boiling water

MAKES & KEEPS
Makes enough for 1 bath. Use right away.

METHOD
Infuse the ingredients together for 10–15 minutes (p.15). Add to a basin containing sufficient hot water for a foot bath: the water should be as hot as comfortable for the feet. Sit with your feet in it for 15–20 mins.

'Beach Hair' Styling Spray for Curls

You can save a lot of money by making your own 'beach hair' spray for that windswept look.

INGREDIENTS
- 500ml/2 cups boiling water
- 4½ tbs Epsom salts
- 1 tbs rosemary tincture (pp.18–19; use 3 tsp rosemary infused in 6 tsp vodka)
- 1 tbs lemon juice
- 2 tsp aloe vera gel
- ½ tsp almond oil
- 10 drops lemon essential oil (optional)

MAKES & KEEPS
Makes about 500ml/2 cups.
Keeps in fridge around 3 months.

METHOD
Mix the ingredients into a spray bottle and spray as much as is required to style your hair.

Citrus Hair Spray

This works well as a hair spray to keep hair in place, but only lasts for a week.

INGREDIENTS
- 2 lemons
- 1 lime
- 500ml/2 cups water (more if required)

MAKES & KEEPS
Makes 250ml/1 cup.
Keeps 1 week in the fridge.

METHOD
Cut up the lemons and lime. Simmer in the water for about 1 hour, keeping the water level up to 250ml/1 cup (half the amount you started with) by adding more as it boils away.

Leave to cool. Strain well and bottle in a spray bottle.

Spray as much as is required to style your hair.

Super Anti-cellulite Oil

Courtesy of Teri Evans

INGREDIENTS
- 4 tbs grapeseed oil
- 7 large fresh ivy leaves
- 1 tsp wheatgerm oil

Essential oils:
- 7 drops juniper
- 3 drops geranium
- 2 drops rosemary

MAKES & KEEPS
Makes 60ml/¼ cup.
Keeps 6 months.

METHOD
Make an infused oil (p.20) with the grapeseed oil and the ivy. Add the wheatgerm oil and essential oils. Bottle.

Massage well into the usual problem areas 1–2 times daily.

Anti-Cold Sore Lip Balm

INGREDIENTS
- 2 tsp cocoa butter
- 2 tsp shea butter
- 2 tsp beeswax
- 4 tsp coconut oil
- 4 tsp St John's Wort Oil (p.83)
- oil from 5 vitamin E capsules (400 IU)
- 10 drops lemon balm essential oil

YOU WILL NEED
- 16 LIPSTICK MOULDS

MAKES & KEEPS
Makes 16 lip balms using lipstick moulds.
Keeps 6 months or more.

METHOD
Melt all the ingredients except the vitamin E and lemon balm oils in a bain-marie. When melted, remove from the heat and add the vitamin E and lemon balm oil and pour into moulds.

Chocolate Bomb Lip Therapy

Courtesy of Monika Ghent

This luscious lip balm heals and protects the delicate skin of your lips.

INGREDIENTS
- 2 tsp beeswax
- 2 tsp cocoa butter
- 2 tsp shea butter
- 20g/¾oz dark cooking chocolate
- 4 tsp olive oil
- oil from 5 vitamin E capsules (400 IU)
- 10 drops peppermint essential oil

YOU WILL NEED
- 16 LIPSTICK MOULDS OR LIP BALM JARS

MAKES & KEEPS
Makes 16 lip balms using lipstick moulds or jars.
Keeps 6 months or more.

METHOD
In a double boiler, melt the beeswax, cocoa butter, shea butter and chocolate. When melted add the olive oil, then take off the heat and add the vitamin E oil.

Lastly, add the peppermint essential oil. Stir well and then put into the lip balm jars or lipstick moulds immediately.

Doux-baiser Lipstick (Sweet Kiss)

Courtesy of Christine Herren-Valette

Protects the lips while adding a touch of colour.

INGREDIENTS
- 1 tsp beeswax
- 4 tsp Heal-all Marigold Oil (p.81)

Essential oils:
- 6 drops rose
- 12 drops rosewood
- tiny pinch of Italian ochre earth (pink)

YOU WILL NEED
- 5/6 LIPSTICK MOULDS

MAKES & KEEPS
Makes 5 or 6 sticks. Keeps 1 year.

METHOD
Melt the beeswax and the marigold oil in a bain-marie. Remove from the heat and add the essential oils.

Mix all the ingredients with either a wooden stick (such as a wooden spoon handle) or a glass stick (not metal or plastic) for 2–3 mins.

Add the Italian ochre earth and stir for a further 1–2 mins to obtain a homogeneous colour. Pour straight away into moulds.

Beetroot Lippy

Vitamin-rich beetroot both conditions and colours your lips.

INGREDIENTS
- 4 tsp St John's Wort Oil (p.83)
- 3 tsp fresh grated beetroot
- 1 tsp beeswax

Essential oils:
- 8 drops orange
- 8 drops lemon

YOU WILL NEED
- 5/6 LIPSTICK MOULDS

MAKES & KEEPS
Makes 5 or 6 sticks.
Keeps 1 year.

METHOD
Pour the St John's Wort Oil over the beetroot. Leave in a covered jar for 3 days, then strain and squeeze out all the oil (wear gloves because the beetroot stains).

Gently melt the beeswax into the beetroot oil. Remove from the heat, stir the essential oils in thoroughly and pour into moulds.

Natural Mascara

Courtesy of Monika Ghent

This mascara isn't waterproof, so is easy to remove with water or vegetable oil.

INGREDIENTS
- 15g/1 tbs white clay (kaolin)
- 0.3g/¼ tsp black mineral oxide
- 2.5ml/½ tsp vegetable glycerine
- 7.5ml/1½ tsp witch hazel
- 10 drops lavender essential oil
- 1 drop oregano essential oil

YOU WILL NEED
- A SYRINGE
- 2 WELL-WASHED MASCARA CASES

MAKES & KEEPS
Makes 2 mascara containers.
Keeps 3 months maximum.

METHOD
Blend all the ingredients well in a small bowl. Using a syringe, insert the mascara into the mascara container. Alternatively, store in a small jar and apply it with an old mascara applicator or eyebrow brush.

SOAP MAKING

You can buy the pure vegetable oil soap needed for many personal care and household cleaning recipes in this book or make your own from scratch. Making soap involves first preparing the lye, then separately warming and mixing an oil component, and finally mixing these. Other ingredients are mostly added later (unless the recipe says otherwise). The recipe for Citrus Oats & Honey Soap (opposite) explains the process in full; others refer back to it and explain the individual differences. Make sure you will not be disturbed, and keep children and animals away. Once underway you cannot stop for some time.

Read 'Key Techniques' on p.21 before commencing.

All these soaps will keep for several years.

> **Caution**
> Have all equipment ready before you start, including safety equipment. Soap making involves handling a dangerous chemical substance, so needs extra caution. It helps to weigh or measure all the ingredients before you start, and have them safely stowed and ready to use.

YOU WILL NEED

- SAFETY: OVERALLS, GLOVES, PROTECTIVE GLASSES OR GOGGLES, HAIR COVERING
- VINEGAR OR LEMON JUICE TO HAND (TO NEUTRALIZE POSSIBLE LYE BURNS)
- DIGITAL SCALES (ACCURATE WEIGHING/MEASURING IS ESSENTIAL)
- STAINLESS STEEL OR ENAMEL SAUCEPAN, WITH A 3–4 LITRES/3–4 QUARTS CAPACITY
- SILICONE OR STAINLESS SPATULA/SPOON
- SMALL STAINLESS STEEL/GLASS/PLASTIC BOWLS
- BUCKET
- MEASURING JUG

The recipes on pages 195 to 198 use a cold process. For cold-process solid soap making you will also need:

- A SUGAR THERMOMETER
- MOULDS – EITHER SILICONE SOAP MOULDS OR A LARGE MOULD THAT YOU WILL LATER CUT INTO BARS – FOR EXAMPLE, A WOODEN BOX LINED WITH PLASTIC

The recipes on pages 198 and 199 use a hot process. For hot-process liquid soap making you will also need:

- A SLOW COOKER (ONE USED FOR SOAP ONLY)
- A HAND-HELD BLENDER (ALSO CALLED A STICK BLENDER, OR IMMERSION BLENDER)
- 1 OR MORE CONTAINERS WITH TIGHT-FITTING LIDS TO STORE 5 LITRES/1 GALLON SOAP

Citrus, Oat & Honey Soap

Courtesy of Emma Warrener

The oats give texture and add a fantastic exfoliant effect.

INGREDIENTS

Lye:
- 295g/10½oz sodium hydroxide
- 900g/30oz water

Oils:
- 615g/21oz coconut oil
- 742g/26oz sunflower oil
- 727g/25oz good-quality olive oil

Extras:
- 200g/1 cup oats
- 150g/almost ½ cup honey
- 100 drops/1 tsp lime essential oil
- 100 drops/1 tsp lemongrass essential oil

MAKES
Makes approx. 30 bars, each weighing 110g/3½oz.

METHOD

Wearing gloves and eye protection, make the lye by carefully pouring the sodium hydroxide crystals into the container holding the water, then leave it out of harm's way to cool to 27–30°C/ 80.6–86°F. (Never pour water on to the lye.)

While this is cooling, gently heat the oils together until the coconut oil is melted and cool to 27–30°C/80.6–86°F.

Carefully pour the lye into the oils and stir with the spatula until you reach 'trace' – this is when you stir and the movement of the spatula creates a line on the top of the mixture – a 'trace' that doesn't disappear. It's a sign that your soap has reached full saponification – when the lye has turned the oils to soap – and indicates your misture is ready. To reach trace usually takes about ½ hour, but soap has its own time scale and it can take much longer! Make sure to stir very thoroughly, all around the sides and the bottom of the pan, and continuously.

When you've achieved a trace, it's time to add the extras (oats, honey and essential oils). It is easiest to do this by putting a small ladle of the mixture in a small bowl, mixing in the extras, then adding this into the main mix and stirring well to ensure they are distributed evenly through the mixture.

Pour the soap into moulds and put in a safe place, away from children in order for it to set for 24 hours. After 24 hours remove from the moulds (wear gloves, as the soap is still caustic) and put it in a dry place to cure for 4–5 weeks.

— *Tip* —

MIXING THE OILS IN A SMALL AMOUNT AS DESCRIBED IS EASIER TO WORK WITH AND ENSURES THEY ARE WELL BLENDED. IT ALSO MEANS YOU CAN EXPERIMENT WITH DIFFERENT ESSENTIAL OILS WITHOUT THE DANGER OF RUINING YOUR WHOLE BATCH OF SOAP, AS SOME WILL REACT DIFFERENTLY.

Bug Off! Insect-repellent Soap

Courtesy of Tanya Smart

INGREDIENTS

Lye:
- 112g/4oz sodium hydroxide
- 362ml/13oz water

Oils:
- 375g/13oz coconut oil
- 300g/10½oz olive oil
- 100g/3½oz cocoa butter
- 50g/2oz shea butter

Essential oils:
- 2 tsp may chang
- 100 drops/1 tsp Virginian cedarwood
- 100 drops/1 tsp juniper
- 50 drops/½ tsp basil

MAKES

Makes 12 bars, each weighing 110g/3½oz.

METHOD

Make as for Citrus, Oat & Honey Soap (p.195). First, prepare the lye and set aside to warm. Then warm the oils. Mix the lye and the oil parts together to trace, before adding the essential oils.

Sugar & Spice Body & Shampoo Bar

Courtesy of Tanya Smart

INGREDIENTS

Lye:
- 112g/4oz sodium hydroxide
- 362ml/13oz water

Oils:
- 375g/13oz coconut oil
- 300g/10½oz olive oil
- 100g/3½oz cocoa butter
- 50g/2oz shea butter

- 1 tbs golden syrup
- 2 tsp jojoba oil

Essential oils:
- 1½ tsp orange
- 100 drops/1 tsp ylang ylang
- 100 drops/1 tsp black pepper
- 50 drops/½ tsp ground cinnamon
- 50 drops/½ tsp ground nutmeg

MAKES

Makes 12 bars, each weighing 110g/3½oz.

METHOD

Make as for Citrus, Oat & Honey Soap (p.195). First, prepare the lye and set aside to warm. Then warm the oils, adding the golden syrup to the mix as it is warming. Mix the lye and the oil parts together to trace, before adding the jojoba oil and essential oils.

Gardeners' Soap for Dirty Nails

Courtesy of Tanya Smart

INGREDIENTS

Lye:
- 112g/4oz sodium hydroxide
- 362ml/13oz water

Oils:
- 375g/13oz coconut oil
- 300g/10½oz olive oil
- 100g/3½oz cocoa butter
- 50g/2oz shea butter

Essential oils:
- 2 tsp clary sage
- 100 drops/1 tsp lavender
- 50 drops/½ tsp rosemary
- 50 drops/½ tsp bay

- 1 tbs coffee, roughly ground
- 1 tsp spirulina powder

MAKES

Makes 12 bars, each weighing 110g/3½oz.

METHOD

Make as for Citrus, Oat & Honey Soap (p.195). First, prepare the lye and set aside to warm. Then warm the oils. Mix the lye and the oil parts together to trace, before adding the essential oils, coffee grounds and spirulina.

Baby Bubbles

Courtesy of Tanya Smart

Gentle and mild soap for sensitive skin.

INGREDIENTS

Lye:
- 112g/4oz sodium hydroxide
- 362ml/13oz water

Oils:
- 375g/13oz coconut oil
- 300g/10½oz olive oil
- 100g/3½oz cocoa butter
- 50g/2oz shea butter

Essential oils:
- 2 tsp may chang
- 100 drops/1 tsp Virginian cedarwood
- 100 drops/1 tsp juniper
- 50 drops/½ tsp basil

- 4 tsp dried lavender flowers
- 1 tbs dried marigold petals

MAKES

Makes 12 bars, each weighing 110g/3½oz.

METHOD

Make as for Citrus, Oat & Honey Soap (p.195). First, prepare the lye and set aside to warm. Then warm the oils. Mix the lye and the oil parts together to trace, before adding the essential oils, lavender flowers and marigold petals.

Luxury Soap

Courtesy of Tanya Smart

INGREDIENTS

Lye:
- 124g/4½oz sodium hydroxide
- 375g/13½oz water

Oils:
- 475g/16¾oz coconut oil
- 300g/10½oz olive oil
- 50g/1¾oz shea butter
- 20g/1oz beeswax

- 1 tbs milk powder (optional)
- 3 tbs honey
- 3 tbs oats

Essential oils:
- 100 drops/1 tsp sandalwood
- 100 drops/1 tsp frankincense
- 100 drops/1 tsp rose
- 100 drops/1 tsp ylang-ylang
- 50 drops/½ tsp patchouli

- 2 tsp castor oil

MAKES

Makes 12 bars, each weighing 110g/3½oz.

METHOD

Make as for Citrus, Oat & Honey Soap (p.195). First, prepare the lye and set aside to warm. Then warm the oils, adding the milk powder, honey and oats as they warm. Make sure the beeswax is completely melted with the other oils. Mix the lye and the oil parts together to trace, before adding the essential oils and castor oil.

Pure Olive Oil Castile Soap

Pure castile soap is made from olive oil using a hot process (p.194). An extremely moisturizing, mild soap, it is kind on the skin.

INGREDIENTS

- 1330g/47oz organic olive oil

Lye:
- 900g/30oz distilled water
- 266g/9.39oz potassium hydroxide

- 2.37 litres/80oz distilled water (separate from the lye)

MAKES & KEEPS

Makes just under 5 litres/1 gallon of liquid soap. Keeps 1 year or more.

METHOD

Put the olive oil in your slow cooker and turn it on to its low setting.

Meanwhile, make the lye. Do this outside if possible, or by an open window. Put the 900g/30oz of water in a large, stainless steel pan. Put on goggles and gloves.

Pour the potassium hydroxide into the water very carefully and slowly, without splashing. (Note: NEVER pour the water into the lye as this is very dangerous.)

Next, pour the lye/water mixture slowly and carefully into the oil in the slow cooker. Stir it with a spoon that can take the heat. The oil will become cloudy.

Stir very carefully without splashing, until you have the 'trace' on the top, as with all soap making. You may need to stir for a long time – a stick blender on slow can take from 5–10 mins to 40 mins or more – and once started you cannot stop.

When you have the 'trace' put the lid on the slow cooker and leave it (still on low) for 20 mins. Every 20 mins or so give it another stir and mix well – don't worry if it separates, as this is normal. Stir well to mix, being careful as it is still corrosive.

BEAUTY, BALMS & PERSONAL CARE

Fairly soon the mixture gets too thick to stir with the blender, so use a spoon or spatula to stir instead. (It's handy to have both.) The mixture starts to resemble very thick mashed potatoes, quite difficult to mix. Continue to stir every 20 mins, until the thick mixture is translucent, though yellowish in colour. It will take up to 12 hours, though the blended soap may be done in 4–5. If you need to, turn off the slow cooker and go to bed for the night, resuming in the morning.

After 4–5 hours, test it by very carefully dissolving 25g/1oz of the mixture into 55g/2oz very hot water in a clear glass container.

Stir it – if it goes milky or cloudy, it needs to cook for longer. If it is clear, it's ready.

When it is ready, carefully weigh the thick paste (wearing gloves) and put it in a large pan. Bring the same quantity of water by weight (500g/16 oz water to every 500g/16 oz paste) almost to the boil and pour on top.

Stir very gently to dissolve. This can take a long time – you need to stir, possibly heat it some more, and stir again. If it keeps forming a whitish layer on top, you need to dilute more – add up to the same amount of water again and heat, stirring gently. Store in large jars.

Though I have used it immediately, it becomes more gentle with time, and I recommend leaving it for 4–6 weeks to 'cure' before use.

Liquid Castile Soap

Nowadays, many blended vegetable oil soaps are called 'castile' or 'Marseille' soap. This blended soap is less moisturizing but more strongly cleansing than the pure olive oil one.

INGREDIENTS
- 565g/20oz olive oil
- 400g/14oz sunflower oil
- 425g/15oz coconut oil

Lye:
- 900g/30oz distilled water
- 270g/9½oz potassium hydroxide

- 2.3 litres/80oz distilled water (separate from the lye)

MAKES & KEEPS
Makes around 5 litres/1 gallon of liquid soap. Keeps 1 year or more.

METHOD
Make as for Pure Olive Oil Castile Soap (left), replace the single quantity of olive oil with the blend of 3 oils (above). These ingredients will take less time to saponify than the Pure Olive Oil Castile Soap, so you'll find you won't be stirring the mixture for as long.

Luxury Moisturizing Handwash

INGREDIENTS
- 2 tsp avocado oil

Essential oils:
- 10 drops chamomile
- 10 drops lavender
- 10 drops neroli

- 1 tsp glycerine
- 2 tbs liquid soap (Pure Olive Oil Castile Soap, pp.198–99, will be the most moisturizing)
- 2 tbs + 2 tsp boiled or distilled water
- 2 tbs + 2 tsp rosewater

MAKES & KEEPS
Makes 125ml/½ cup.
Keeps effective at least 3 months.

METHOD
Whisk the avocado oil and essential oils into the glycerine. Slowly mix in the rest of the ingredients. Pour into a hand-soap dispenser. Shake from time to time.

Lavender Handwash

INGREDIENTS
- 2 tsp Lavender-infused Oil (p.73)
- 30 drops lavender essential oil
- 1 tsp glycerine
- 2 tbs Liquid Castile Soap (p.199)
- 2 tbs + 2 tsp boiled or distilled water
- 2 tbs + 2 tsp lavender water

MAKES & KEEPS
Makes 125ml/½ cup.
Keeps effective at least 3 months.

METHOD
Whisk the Lavender-infused Oil and essential oil into the glycerine. Then make and use as for Luxury Moisturizing Handwash (above).

Mandarin Handwash

INGREDIENTS
- 2 tsp infused lemon oil (p.20)

Essential oils:
- 20 drops mandarin
- 20 drops orange
- 10 drops tea tree

- 1 tsp glycerine
- 2 tbs Liquid Castile Soap (p.199)
- 2 tbs + 2 tsp boiled or distilled water
- 2 tbs + 2 tsp orange-flower or witch hazel water

MAKES & KEEPS
Makes 125ml/½ cup.
Keeps at least 3 months.

METHOD
Make as for Luxury Moisturizing Handwash (left).

Antibacterial Liquid Handwash

This combines the bacteria-zapping actions of witch hazel, tea tree, lavender and thyme to make a powerful soap with a fresh odour.

INGREDIENTS
- 2 tsp almond oil

Essential oils:
- 20 drops tea tree
- 20 drops lavender
- 10 drops thyme

- 1 tsp glycerine
- 2 tbs Liquid Castile Soap (p.199)
- 3 tbs + 1 tsp boiled or distilled water
- 2 tbs distilled witch hazel

MAKES & KEEPS
Makes 125ml/½ cup.
Keeps at least 3 months.

METHOD
Make as for Luxury Moisturizing Handwash (left).

BEAUTY, BALMS & PERSONAL CARE

Moisturizing Working Hand Scrub

Courtesy of Teri Evans

INGREDIENTS
- 100g/5½ tbs fine sea salt
- up to 100ml/6¾ tbs sunflower oil

Essential oils:
- 10 drops lemon
- 15 drops lavender
- 10 drops geranium

MAKES & KEEPS
Makes 200g/¾ cup.
Keeps 6 months.

METHOD
Put the salt in a bowl and trickle enough sunflower oil into it to make a thick paste. Add the essential oils and stir well. Store in a jar.

Wet your hands and massage about 1 tsp of the scrub gently into your hands. Rinse off. The oil should leave your hands feeling soft.

Clay Soap Alternative

A simple clay wash for your face, hands, body and hair. Use any fine clay earth, such as Tilak from India or Rassoul Clay from Morocco, or whatever you have locally (if you dig up your own, be sure to carefully sieve and filter it to remove stones).

INGREDIENTS
- 1–3 tsp fine clay
- 1–3 tsp rosewater

MAKES & KEEPS
1 wash.
Make and use same day.

METHOD
Wet your skin, take a little clay powder and rub it over your skin, applying more water as needed. Allow it to stay on the skin for a few minutes, and wash off. For a lovely face wash, mix the clay with a little rosewater and then apply.

Psoriasis Skin Scrub

Courtesy of Lynn Rawlinson

Use this gentle alternative to soap in the bath or shower to help with de-scaling.

INGREDIENTS
- 100g/½ cup coconut oil
- 50g/¼ cup Lavender-infused Oil (p.73)
- 50g/⅓ cup oatmeal
- 25 drops/¼ tsp helichynum essential oil

MAKES & KEEPS
Makes 200g/almost 1 cup.
Keeps 1 year.

METHOD
Melt the coconut and lavender oils in a double boiler or bain-marie. Leave until it starts to cool. Whisk until it is tepid and the oil is starting to solidify. Blend in the oatmeal and add the essential oil.

Before bathing, apply skin scrub to flannel and lightly rub over the body. Soak in the bath or shower, rubbing the skin while in the water. Towel dry leaving the skin soft and smooth.

Anti-ageing Skin Scrub

Courtesy of Lynn Rawlinson

INGREDIENTS
- 100g/½ cup coconut oil
- 50g/¼ cup Lavender-infused Oil (p.73)
- 50g/⅓ cup oatmeal

Essential oils:
- 15 drops frankincense
- 4 drops geranium
- 4 drops neroli light
- 10 drops lavender

MAKES & KEEPS
Makes 200g/almost 1 cup.
Keeps 1 year.

METHOD
Make and use as for Psoriasis Skin Scrub (above).

Healing Skin Scrub

Courtesy of Lynn Rawlinson

INGREDIENTS
- 100g/½ cup coconut oil
- 50g/¼ cup Lavender-infused Oil (p.73)
- 50g/⅓ cup oatmeal

Essential oils:
- 25 drops/¼ tsp lavender
- 10 drops geranium

MAKES & KEEPS
Makes 200g/almost 1 cup.
Keeps 1 year.

METHOD
Make and use as for Psoriasis Skin Scrub (p.201).

Coconut Scrub for Blemishes

Courtesy of Lynn Rawlinson

INGREDIENTS
- 100g/½ cup coconut oil
- 50g/¼ cup Lavender-infused Oil (p.73)
- 50g/⅓ cup oatmeal

Essential oils:
- 30 drops lavender
- 10 drops chamomile

MAKES & KEEPS
Makes 200g/almost 1 cup.
Keeps 1 year.

METHOD
Make and use as for Psoriasis Skin Scrub (p.201).

Soapwort Shampoo for Dark Hair

Courtesy of Teri Evans

This leaves your hair so soft and glossy you will love it!

INGREDIENTS
Dried herbs:
- 10g/½oz Irish moss seaweed
- 25g/1oz soapwort root, coarsely ground
- 10g/½oz sage
- 150ml/⅔ cup boiling water

MAKES & KEEPS
Enough for 1–2 applications.
Use within 3 days.

METHOD
Crumble the Irish moss and mix in with the other dry ingredients. Put in a jug and pour on the boiling water. Leave to cool stirring occasionally. Strain through muslin, pushing it through to leave a greenish slime.

Use like normal shampoo, but don't expect it to foam. Rinse well.

Note: avoid getting it in your eyes – it will sting a lot.

Soapwort Shampoo for Blondes

Courtesy of Teri Evans

INGREDIENTS
Dried herbs:
- 10g/½oz Irish moss seaweed
- 25g/1oz soapwort root, coarsely ground
- 10g/½oz chamomile
- 150ml/⅔ cup boiling water

MAKES & KEEPS
Enough for 1–2 applications.
Use within 3 days.

METHOD
Make and use as for Soapwort Shampoo for Dark Hair (above).

Soapwort Shampoo for Redheads

Courtesy of Teri Evans

INGREDIENTS
Dried herbs:
- 10g/½oz Irish moss seaweed
- 25g/1oz soapwort root, coarsely ground
- 10g/½oz marigold petals
- 150ml/⅔ cup boiling water

MAKES & KEEPS
Enough for 1–2 applications.
Use within 3 days.

METHOD
Make and use as for Soapwort Shampoo for Dark Hair (left).

Red Clover Mild Shampoo

For normal hair, and also good for children.

INGREDIENTS
- 250ml/1 cup boiling distilled water
- 10g/¼ cup fresh red clover flowers (or 7g/¼oz dried)
- 1 tsp apricot kernel oil or almond oil
- 2 drops Roman chamomile essential oil
- 2 tbs liquid soap, castile if liked (p.199), or any kind of shampoo base

MAKES & KEEPS
Makes approx. 260ml/just over 1 cup.
Keeps up to 2 months.

METHOD
Make and use as for Comfrey & Elder Shampoo for Dry Hair (right).

Comfrey & Elder Shampoo for Dry Hair

Courtesy of Karen Stephenson

INGREDIENTS
- 10g/¼ cup fresh comfrey root (or 7g/¼oz dried)
- 10g/¼ cup fresh elder flowers (or 7g/¼oz dried)
- 250ml/1 cup boiling distilled water

Essential oils:
- 6 drops neroli
- 6 drops lavender
- 1 tsp apricot kernel oil or almond oil
- 2 tbs liquid soap, castile if liked (p.199), or any type of shampoo base

MAKES & KEEPS
Makes approx. 260ml/just over 1 cup.
Keeps up to 2 months.

METHOD
Infuse the herbs with the boiling water for 20 mins (p.15). Strain and mix the essential oils with the apricot kernel or almond oil, then mix thoroughly with the soap or shampoo base. Gently mix with the infused herbs.

Shake gently before each use.

Willow Shampoo for Oily Hair

Courtesy of Karen Stephenson

INGREDIENTS
- 250ml/1 cup boiling distilled water
- 10g/⅓oz dried white willow bark
- 10g/⅓oz dried lemongrass (or 10g/¼ cup freshly grated)
- 1 tsp apricot kernel oil or almond oil

Essential oils:
- 6 drops bergamot
- 6 drops cedarwood
- 2 tbs liquid soap, castile if liked (p.199), or any kind of shampoo base

MAKES & KEEPS
Makes approx. 260ml/just over 1 cup.
Keeps up to 2 months.

METHOD
Make and use as described for Comfrey & Elder Shampoo for Dry Hair (p.203).

Burdock Anti-dandruff Shampoo

Courtesy of Karen Stephenson

INGREDIENTS
- 250ml/1 cup boiling distilled water
- 10g/¼ cup grated fresh burdock root (or 7g/¼oz dried)
- 10g/¼ cup fresh chamomile flowers (or 7g/¼oz dried)
- 1 tsp apricot kernel oil or almond oil
- 12 drops rosemary essential oil
- 2 tbs liquid soap, castile if liked (p.199), or any kind of shampoo base

MAKES & KEEPS
Makes approx. 260ml/just over 1 cup.
Keeps up to 2 months.

METHOD
Make and use as described for Comfrey & Elder Shampoo for Dry Hair (p.203).

Cornflour & Rosemary Dry Shampoo

A quick alternative to washing your hair.

INGREDIENTS
- 1 tbs dried rosemary, ground to a powder
- 150g/1 cup cornflour

MAKES & KEEPS
Makes approx. 150g/1 cup.
Keeps at least a year if kept dry.

METHOD
Thoroughly mix the rosemary and cornflour.
Store in a sugar shaker for easy use.
Apply a little of the powder to your hair roots. Rub it in well with your fingers, then brush it very thoroughly to remove the grease.

— *Tip* —

ADD A COUPLE OF DROPS OF AN ESSENTIAL OIL TO YOUR SHAMPOO FOR A STRONGER FRAGRANCE.

Nettle & Sage Shampoo for Greying Hair

Use this to slow down greying.

INGREDIENTS
- 250ml/1 cup boiling distilled water
- 10g/⅓oz dried nettles
- 10g/⅓oz dried sage
- 1 tsp almond oil
- 4 drops rosemary essential oil
- 2 tbs liquid soap, castile if liked (p.199), or any kind of shampoo base

MAKES & KEEPS
Makes approx. 260ml/just over 1 cup. Keeps up to 2 months.

METHOD
Make and use as described for Comfrey & Elder Shampoo for Dry Hair (p.203).

Hair Mud

Courtesy of Teri Evans

Suitable for all hair types except very dry. Either use it as a shampoo or leave on for 20 mins as a deep cleansing hair pack. Your hair feels incredibly clean after use.

INGREDIENTS
- ½ tbs rhassoul mud powder (this is a Moroccan mud from the Atlas Mountains but you can actually use any sort of clay)
- 2 tbs herbal infusion (p.15): chamomile for blonde, marigold for red, nettle for brown, sage or black tea for black

MAKES & KEEPS
Enough for 1–2 applications. Keep in the fridge and use within 1 week.

METHOD
Mix the mud and herbal infusion well. Leave it to stand for 5 mins. Stir again and add more infusion if needed.

Massage the clay through your hair like a shampoo. Leave for a few minutes, then rinse off thoroughly.

Orange, Lime & Grapefruit Conditioner

Courtesy of Emma Warrener

INGREDIENTS

Oil fraction:
- 1 tsp coconut oil
- 2 tbs emulsifying wax
- 1 tsp grapeseed oil

- 125ml/½ cup water (or floral water, or herbal infusion, p.15)
- 1 tsp glycerine
- oil from 2 vitamin E capsules (400 IU)

Essential oils:
- 30 drops sweet orange
- 30 drops lime
- 30 drops grapefruit

MAKES & KEEPS

Makes approx. 150ml/just under ⅔ cup.
Keeps up to 1 year.

METHOD

Gently heat the oil fraction in a double boiler with the water (or floral water or herbal infusion) in the bottom pan. When the oils are melted, remove the pan from the heat and leave to cool for 5 mins.

Meanwhile, measure the warmed water and top up to 125ml/½ cup. Add the glycerine to the water and stir thoroughly.

Slowly add the water mixture to the oil mixture, whisking continuously. The mixture will thicken up as it cools down. Once all of the water has been added mix in the vitamin E oil and essential oils.

Leave to cool completely, whisking now and then to ensure that the liquid doesn't separate.

Store in a recycled plastic shampoo/conditioner bottle for ease of use.

Apply to clean, wet hair, leave on for 2–4 mins, then rinse thoroughly.

Nit-deterring Conditioner

INGREDIENTS

Oil fraction:
- 1 tsp coconut oil
- 2 tbs emulsifying wax
- 1 tsp neem oil

- 125ml/½ cup water (or lavender water or quassia infusion, p.15)
- 1 tsp glycerine
- oil from 2 vitamin E capsules (400 IU)

Essential oils:
- 30 drops tea tree
- 40 drops lavender
- 20 drops thyme

MAKES & KEEPS

Makes approx. 150ml/just under ⅔ cup.
Keeps 1–2 months.

METHOD

Make and use as for Orange, Lime & Grapefruit Conditioner (left).

— *Variation* —

VARY THE ESSENTIAL OILS TO SUIT YOUR NEEDS. SEE THE HERBAL INFUSIONS AND OILS USED IN THE SHAMPOO RECIPES FOR INSPIRATION. IF YOU ADD A HERBAL INFUSION IN PLACE OF THE WATER, THE CONDITIONER WILL ONLY KEEP UP TO 1–2 MONTHS.

— *Tip* —

PURE, NATURAL YOGURT IS A GOOD CONDITIONER. APPLY TO HAIR AS YOU WOULD A SHOP-BOUGHT CONDITIONER. ONCE EVERY 1–2 WEEKS USE A DEEP TREATMENT, SUCH AS HAIR MILK OR OIL.

All-natural Hot Oil Hair Treatment

INGREDIENTS
- 250ml/1 cup olive oil
- 3 tbs dried rosemary leaves

MAKES & KEEPS
Makes 250ml/1 cup.
Keeps 6 months.

METHOD
Make an infused oil with the rosemary and olive oil (p.20). Wash your hair and towel dry. Apply 2–5 tbs of the oil to your hair and massage it. Put a plastic cap on and wrap your head in a towel. After 45–90 mins, wash your hair with a gentle shampoo.

Use weekly or less, as required.

Tropical Hair Milk

Courtesy of Teri Evans

This alternative to a hot oil treatment is less greasy but deeply conditioning for the hair. It smells deliciously tropical. Suitable for all hair types.

INGREDIENTS
- 100ml/just under ½ cup coconut milk
- 7 drops lemon balm oil
- 4 drops ylang-ylang essential oil

MAKES & KEEPS
Enough for 1 application.
Use immediately.

METHOD
Combine all the ingredients in a jug.

Massage into your hair and leave on for 10–20 mins. Wash with a gentle shampoo.

You can use this treatment up to once a week, as desired.

Sweet Rose Hair Oil

A sweet-smelling hair oil, very simple to make.

INGREDIENTS
- 15g/½oz dried rose petals or buds
- 200g/approx. 1 cup coconut oil
- 4–8 drops rose (or rose geranium) essential oil

MAKES & KEEPS
Makes 200g/approx 1 cup.
Keeps 6–12 months.

METHOD
Place the roses and the coconut oil in a double boiler. Heat on a very low heat for 2–3 hours. Strain, add the essential oil and pour into a jar.

Melt and use as described for All-natural Hot Oil Hair Treatment (above). Alternatively, apply a little to your fingers and massage into the ends of your hair daily to moisturize.

Hair Growth Tonic

Courtesy of Johanna Herzog

Helps to stimulate and warm the scalp, so helping hair growth.

INGREDIENTS
- 500ml/2 cups vodka
- 125ml/½ cup water
- 2 handfuls of fresh young birch leaves (collected in spring), shredded
- 2 handfuls of fresh nettle leaves and roots
- 1–2 fresh burdock roots, chopped
- 1 vanilla pod (optional)

MAKES & KEEPS
Makes approx. 500ml/2 cups.
Keeps 1 year.

METHOD
Mix in a covered jar and leave for 2 weeks, then strain as for any tincture (pp.18–19).

Dilute a little of the tonic with the same amount of water and massage into the scalp daily.

Rosemary Vinegar

Helps to promote hair growth as a hair rinse, and to improve the memory and circulation as a drink. It has a fresh smell and some antiseptic properties, so is also useful in cleaning products.

INGREDIENTS
- 30g/1 cup rosemary flowering tops
- 500ml/2 cups Apple Cider Vinegar (p.165)

MAKES & KEEPS
Makes 450ml/almost 2 cups.
Keeps at least 2 years.

METHOD
Make as for vinegars (pp.163–65).

For use on hair, dilute 1 part to 2 parts water. Apply on wet hair after washing/conditioning as a final rinse. You can also put it in a spray bottle and spray on to wet hair.

Hair & Herbal Vinegars

Herbal vinegars when used as a hair rinse will encourage shine and help restore your hair's protective acid pH. Different vinegars can be used for different effect. Try nettle and rosemary for promoting thickness and increased hair growth, or rosemary and a few drops of tea tree oil to treat dandruff, or sage to darken greying hair.

BEAUTY, BALMS & PERSONAL CARE

Cinnamint Toothpaste

Courtesy of Monika Ghent

To whiten the teeth and strengthen and heal gums.

INGREDIENTS
- 2 tsp bicarbonate of soda
- 2 tbs white clay (kaolin)
- 1 tbs arrowroot powder
- ½ tsp vitamin C powder
- 1 tsp ground cinnamon
- up to 1½ tsp pure liquid soap (castile soap, especially Dr Bronner's, is recommended)
- 15–20 drops peppermint essential oil

Tinctures (pp.18–19):
- 30–50 drops stevia
- 1 tsp echinacea
- 1 tsp sage
- 1 tsp 3 per cent hydrogen peroxide (naturally whitens teeth)

MAKES & KEEPS
Makes approx. 50ml/just under ¼ cup.
Keeps at least 1 year.

METHOD
Combine all the ingredients in a jar and stir well. Slowly add a little water to make a paste, and store.

Use as you would any toothpaste.

Teri's Tooth Powder

Courtesy of Teri Evans

A very simple and effective tooth powder.

INGREDIENTS
- 1 tbs arrowroot
- 1 tsp sea salt
- ½ tsp bicarbonate of soda
- 2 drops peppermint or cinnamon essential oil

YOU WILL NEED
- A PESTLE AND MORTAR

MAKES & KEEPS
Makes 4½ tsp.
Keeps at least 1 year.

METHOD
Mix the ingredients together well. Pound to a dry paste with the pestle and mortar and store.

Use as you would any toothpaste.

— Variation —

ADD 2 DROPS OF CLOVE OIL TO THIS TOOTH POWDER FOR A STRONGLY ANTISEPTIC EFFECT.

Handwritten note:

CLAY TOOTHPASTE

3 tbsp coconut oil
3 tbsp bentonite clay
2 tbsp filtered water
10 drops peppermint oil
+
1 tbsp bicarb. soda

Medicated Tooth Powder for Gum Disease

INGREDIENTS
- ½ tsp ground myrrh
- ½ tsp ground cloves
- 4 tsp bicarbonate of soda
- 1 tsp salt
- 3 tsp gram (chickpea) flour

MAKES & KEEPS
Makes 3 tbs.
Keeps at least 1 year.

METHOD
Combine all the ingredients, mixing well. Store in small airtight jars.

Use a small sprinkle, apply as any toothpaste. Used daily, this amount could last 1–3 months.

Medicinal Mouthwash & Gargle

Helps to treat gum disease, mouth and throat infections.

INGREDIENTS

Tinctures (pp.18–19):
- 20ml/4 tsp myrrh
- 20ml/4 tsp cloves
- 20ml/4 tsp peppermint
- 20ml/4 tsp sage
- 20ml/4 tsp horse chestnut (conker)

Essential oils:
- 1 drop lavender
- 1 drop geranium
- 1 drop eucalyptus

MAKES & KEEPS
Makes 100ml/½ cup.
Keeps 2 years or more.

METHOD
Mix the ingredients together in a bottle.

Shake before use. Dilute ½ tsp in 2 tbs warm water. Use to gargle or mouthwash twice daily.

Sage & Lavender Deodorant

Courtesy of Teri Evans

A floral scent that women may prefer.

INGREDIENTS
- 2 tsp dried sage
- 2 tbs + 2 tsp witch hazel
- 3 tsp fresh cleavers (2 tsp dried)
- 1 tbs vodka
- 1 tsp benzoin (Friar's Balsam) tincture

Essential oils:
- 5 drops sage
- 5 drops lavender

YOU WILL NEED
60ML/2FL.OZ SPRAY BOTTLE

MAKES & KEEPS
Makes 50ml/almost ¼ cup.
Keeps 3–6 months.

METHOD
Leave the sage to infuse in the witch hazel for 2 weeks, and the cleavers to infuse in the vodka for 2 weeks (p.18). Strain and press both, then combine. Add all the other ingredients and mix in a bottle with a spray top. Shake well.

Shake before use and use as a normal deodorant. Men may prefer it without the lavender: simply add sage oil in place of the lavender.

Handwritten note:

TRASH IS FOR TOSSERS!

2 TBSP ARROWROOT POWDER
1 TBSP BAKING SODA
1 TBSP COCONUT OIL
1 TBSP SHEA BUTTER
10 DROPS ESSENTIAL OIL

X 4-5 for big batch

BEAUTY, BALMS & PERSONAL CARE

Citrus Fresh Deodorant

Courtesy of Teri Evans

A fresh smell that men may prefer.

INGREDIENTS
- 2 tsp dried sage
- 2 tbs + 2 tsp witch hazel
- 3 tsp fresh cleavers (2 tsp dried)
- 1 tbs vodka
- 1 tsp benzoin (Friar's Balsam) tincture

Essential oils:
- 5 drops lemongrass
- 5 drops tangerine

YOU WILL NEED
· 60ML/2FL.OZ SPRAY BOTTLE

MAKES & KEEPS
Makes 50ml/just under ¼ cup.
Keeps 3–6 months.

METHOD
Make as for Sage & Lavender Deodorant (opposite).

Sandalwood Deodorant

Courtesy of Teri Evans

A musky and sexy fragrance for men and women.

INGREDIENTS
- 2 tsp dried sage
- 2 tbs + 2 tsp witch hazel
- 3 tsp fresh cleavers (2 tsp dried)
- 1 tbs vodka
- 1 tsp benzoin (Friar's balsam) tincture

Essential oils:
- 5 drops sage
- 5 drops sandalwood

YOU WILL NEED
· 60ML/2FL.OZ SPRAY BOTTLE

MAKES & KEEPS
Makes 50ml/just under ¼ cup.
Keeps 3–6 months.

METHOD
Make as for Sage & Lavender Deodorant (opposite).

Tea Tree & Lemon Deodorant Powder

INGREDIENTS
- 120g/1 cup white clay (kaolin)
- 40g/¼ cup bicarbonate of soda
- 40g/1½oz arrowroot

Essential oils:
- 20 drops tea tree
- 20 drops lemon

MAKES & KEEPS
Makes 200g/1½ cups.
Keeps 1–2 years in an airtight container.

METHOD
Combine all the dry ingredients in a bowl. Slowly add the essential oils, stirring continuously. Sieve the powder before storing.

[Handwritten note at top:] FOR THE LITTLE POTS:
3 tsp clay
1 tsp bicarb.
1 tsp arrowroot
Same quantity of oils

Lavender & Sage Deodorant Powder

Courtesy of Monika Ghent

This very effective, body-friendly, underarm deodorant can also be used as baby powder. Men may prefer it without the lavender oil.

INGREDIENTS

- 120g/4oz white clay (kaolin)
- 40g/¼ cup bicarbonate of soda
- 40g/1½oz arrowroot

Essential oils:
- 20 drops lavender
- 20 drops sage

MAKES & KEEPS

Makes 200g/1½ cups.
Keeps 1–2 years.

METHOD

Mix all the dry ingredients well in a bowl. Slowly drip in the essential oils, stirring constantly throughout. Place the sieve over a second bowl and pour the deodorant into it. Shake the sieve until all the powder has passed through it.

You will be left with little balls of powder and essential oil. Using your fist, gently rub your hand around the sieve to break up these balls so that they pass through. Repeat the process twice more. Then transfer the mixture into one or more glass jars.

Apply a dusting of the powder after washing and drying.

Luxury Shaving Cream for Women

INGREDIENTS

Oil fraction:
- 60ml/4 tbs sweet almond oil (or apricot oil or jojoba oil)
- 10g/2 tbs shea butter or cocoa butter

Water fraction:
- 350ml/1½ cups spring water/filtered water
- 1 tsp bicarbonate of soda
- 4 tbs Liquid Castile Soap (p.199)
- 60ml/¼ cup honey
- 60ml/¼ cup aloe vera gel

Essential oils:
- 5 drops rose
- 5 drops jasmine

MAKES & KEEPS

Makes about 500ml/2 cups.
Keeps at least 3 months.

METHOD

Heat the oil and butter in a double boiler for a few minutes until it looks clear.

Remove the pan and leave to cool. Use the lower pan of the double boiler to heat. Gently heat the water, bicarbonate of soda and liquid soap. Stir until they are completely dissolved and mixed, then add the honey and aloe vera and mix them in.

Slowly mix this mixture into the oils, a little bit at a time. Stir continuously.

Finally, add the essential oils and blend for a few minutes. Then leave to stand for a few minutes and blend again. Pour into jars.

Massage a little into the skin before shaving.

Moisturizing Shaving Cream for Men

INGREDIENTS

Oil fraction:
- 60ml/4 tbs sweet almond oil (or apricot oil or jojoba oil)
- 10g/2 tbs shea butter

Water fraction:
- 350ml/1½ cups spring water/filtered water
- 1 tsp bicarbonate of soda
- 4 tbs Liquid Castile Soap (p.199)
- 120ml/¼ cup aloe vera gel

Essential oils:
- 4 drops pine
- 5 drops rosemary

MAKES & KEEPS

Makes about 500ml/2 cups.
Keeps at least 3 months.

METHOD

Make and use as for Luxury Shaving Cream for Women (opposite), adding the aloe vera when you would have added aloe vera and honey.

Tree Power Antiseptic Aftershave

This very simple aftershave is antiseptic and strongly astringent.

INGREDIENTS
- 20 drops tea tree essential oil
- 120ml/½ cup distilled witch hazel

MAKES & KEEPS

Makes 120ml/about ½ cup.
Keeps 1–2 years.

METHOD

Mix the ingredients and store.

Apply a little to skin after shaving.

Green Dragon Shaving Oil

Courtesy of Alaina Mecklenburgh

INGREDIENTS
- 80ml/⅓ cup almond oil
- 4 tsp glycerine

Essential oils:
- 20 drops eucalyptus
- 20 drops lavender
- 50 drops/½ tsp peppermint

MAKES & KEEPS

Makes 100ml/just under ½ cup.
Keeps at least 6 months.

METHOD

Combine all the ingredients and store in a glass bottle.

Shake before use. Wet your face, put 5–6 drops on your hands and apply to skin. Shave as usual.

Herby Aftershave

INGREDIENTS
- 2 tbs rosemary leaves (fresh or dry)
- 2 tbs lavender flowers (fresh or dry)
- 2 tbs chamomile flowers (fresh or dry)
- 60ml/¼ cup spring water
- 60ml/¼ cup vodka
- 4 tbs witch hazel
- 1 tbs olive oil

MAKES & KEEPS

Makes about 150ml/almost ⅔ cup.
Keeps 6 months–1 year.

METHOD

Mix everything together except for the olive oil. Make a tincture (pp.18–19). After straining and pressing out the liquid, add the olive oil and bottle.

Shake before each use.

Splash a little on to the skin after shaving.

VARIOUS ODDITIES

Everything we need comes from plants – and some things we don't need too! From ink to car wax and some weird and wonderful things in between, this section contains a miscellany of useful recipes I have concocted and gathered over the years.

Blue-purple Ink

INGREDIENTS
- 2 handfuls of ripe elderberries (or bilberries/huckleberries)
- 4 tbs vinegar
- 2.5ml/½ tsp benzoin (Friar's Balsam) tincture or myrrh tincture
- 5 drops thyme or rosemary essential oil
- 1 tsp gum arabic

MAKES & KEEPS
Makes about 60ml/¼ cup.
Keeps around 6 months.

METHOD
Simmer the berries in the vinegar, mashing with a potato masher and stirring to prevent burning, for 15 mins. Strain and press through muslin to get all the juice out (wear gloves as this juice seriously stains).

Mix the other ingredients with the dye/vinegar mixture and bottle.

Use the ink for painting or for writing with a dipping pen and inkwell.

Brown Ink

Courtesy of Teri Evans

INGREDIENTS
- 6–8 whole walnuts, gathered from the ground when blackened with age
- 125ml/½ cup water
- 125ml/½ cup vinegar
- 5ml/1 tsp benzoin (Friar's Balsam) tincture or myrrh tincture
- 5 drops thyme or rosemary essential oil
- 1 tsp gum arabic for each 60ml/¼ cup of dye

MAKES & KEEPS
Makes about 60ml/¼ cup.
Keeps up to 1 year.

METHOD
Simmer the walnut in just enough water to cover for 30 mins–1 hour, topping up with the vinegar as the water boils away. You should end up with 60–120ml/¼–½ cup of dark brown liquid.

Strain the liquid and press through muslin (use gloves and take care as this dye will seriously stain). Mix the other ingredients with the liquid and bottle.

Use as for Blue-purple Ink (left).

Rose Petal Beads

Courtesy of Kamala Todd

The original Rosary prayer beads.

INGREDIENTS
- 2½ litres/2½ quarts fragrant, fresh rose petals
- spring water (variable amount)

YOU WILL NEED
- IRON POT OR CAULDRON

KEEPS
Well-made beads can last over 100 years!

METHOD
Place the rose petals in a little spring water in the iron cauldron and cover with a lid. Gently simmer (never boil hard as the essential oils will be lost) for 5 hours a day for up to 5 days. Add more water as required to stop the rose petals drying out or burning.

Strain and press the liquid through a muslin cloth to leave a thick, smooth, black paste. Roll the paste into bead shapes using your hands (they shrink to ¼–½ of the size when dry).

Place the beads on a plate and leave in a dry, warm place (away from direct sunlight) for 5–10 days to dry. Roll each day to get a dense, smooth, round bead. Before they are completely dry, push a thick needle or skewer through the middle.

Store fully dried beads in glass jars. Do not let the beads get wet.

Waterproofing Mix for Canvas

Courtesy of Teri Evans

INGREDIENTS
- 225ml/1 cup soya, grapeseed or almond oil
- 115ml/½ cup turpentine

MAKES & KEEPS
Makes 340ml/1½ cups.
Keeps at least 1 year.

METHOD
Mix together and store in a cool place.

To waterproof, paint 2–3 coats on to dry canvas.

Lemon Boot Polish

Courtesy of Tony Haslegrave

INGREDIENTS
- 5 tsp beeswax
- 80ml/¼ cup + 2 tsp turpentine
- 1 tbs linseed oil
- 20 drops lemon essential oil

MAKES & KEEPS
Makes 120g/½ cup.
Keeps for years.

METHOD
Heat the beeswax, turpentine and linseed oil together until the wax melts, being careful not to put it on too high a flame or it will catch fire. Add the lemon essential oil, then pour it into tins while still liquid.

THE RECIPES

Walnut Protection Remedy

Courtesy of Lucy Harmer

Helps to relieve the stress of moving and to protect if you feel unsettled or under attack.

INGREDIENTS
- 15 green walnuts, cut into 6–8 pieces
- 500ml/2 cups brandy

MAKES & KEEPS
Makes 500ml/2 cups.
Keeps for years.

METHOD
Macerate the walnuts in the brandy for 6 weeks in a dark place. Stir every 6 days. Strain and bottle as for tinctures (pp.18–19).

To use, half-fill a small dropper bottle with the remedy and top it up with spring water. Take 3–5 drops 3 times daily whenever you feel vulnerable.

Sage Smudge Stick

Courtesy of Lucy Harmer

Smudging, which originates in Native American traditions, is a great way to cleanse a space, home or office. Most smudge sticks are made of sage because it is such a great purifier.

INGREDIENTS
- several small stems fresh sage, about 15–38cm/6–15in long

YOU WILL NEED
- THIN STRING OR COTTON YARN ABOUT 1.5M/5FT LONG

MAKES & KEEPS
Makes 1 stick.
Keeps 1–2 years.

METHOD
Lay the sage stems together so that all the cut ends are on the same side.

Wind the string or cotton tightly around the stems, leaving 5cm/2in of loose string or cotton where you began. Next, wind the string along the length of the bundle until you reach the leafy end. Return to the stalk end, thus creating a criss-cross pattern.

When you get back to the stems, tie the remainder of the string or cotton to the 5cm/2in loose piece you left at the beginning.

Hang the bundle up to dry in a dry place for 3–7 days.

When your smudge stick has dried, you can light the leafy end. Allow it to smoulder and send the smoke around a person, an object or your home to cleanse and purify. Snuff the sage out by pressing the stick down on a plate or small bowl – do not extinguish with water as it is then really difficult to light again.

VARIOUS ODDITIES

Sage & Lavender Smudge Stick

Courtesy of Lucy Harmer

Use to increase mental energy and feel uplifted.

INGREDIENTS
- 5 stems fresh sage, about 15–38cm/6–15in long
- 5 stems fresh sage, about 15–20cm/6–8in long
- 5 stems fresh lavender, about 15–20cm/6–8in long

YOU WILL NEED
- THIN STRING OR COTTON YARN ABOUT 1.5M/5FT LONG

MAKES & KEEPS
Makes 1 stick.
Keeps 1–2 years.

METHOD
Make as for the Sage Smudge Stick (opposite).

— *Variation* —

ADD A LITTLE FRESH MUGWORT TO THIS BUNDLE FOR A MORE HEALING VIBRATION.

Protection Smudge Stick

Courtesy of Lucy Harmer

Use to clear out and cleanse a space from all negative energy and outside influences.

INGREDIENTS
- 3 stems fresh rosemary, about 15–38cm/6–15in long
- 3 stems fresh lavender, about 15–38cm/6–15in long
- 3 stems fresh juniper, about 15–38cm/6–15in long

YOU WILL NEED
- THIN STRING OR COTTON YARN ABOUT 1.5M/5FT LONG

MAKES & KEEPS
Makes 1 stick.
Keeps 1–2 years.

METHOD
Make as for the Sage Smudge Stick (opposite).

Herbal House Cleansing Stick

Courtesy of Lucy Harmer

An ancient European technique for clearing domestic space.

INGREDIENTS
- 500ml/2 cups spring water
- 3 large pinches of salt
- 2 sprigs fresh mint
- 2 sprigs fresh rosemary
- 2 sprigs fresh marjoram

MAKES & KEEPS
Makes enough for 1 use.
Use immediately.

METHOD
Pour the water into a bowl and add the salt.

Weave the herb sprigs together to make a thick loose stick.

Dip the stick in the salt water. Sprinkle around the inside and outside of the home.

Happy Home Charm

Courtesy of Lucy Harmer

A traditional European charm.

INGREDIENTS
- pinch of dried rue
- 2 oak leaves
- 3 dead bumblebees (which have died naturally)

YOU WILL NEED
- A SMALL POUCH OF NATURAL CLOTH

MAKES & KEEPS
Makes 1 charm.
Keeps 1 year.

METHOD
Put the ingredients into the pouch, thinking of your goal. Hang the pouch next to the front door.

House Protection Charm

Courtesy of Lucy Harmer

INGREDIENTS
- 1 tsp dried vervain
- 1 tsp dill seeds
- 1 tsp dried rosemary leaves
- 1 tsp dried bay leaves
- 1 tsp dried St John's wort
- 1 tsp juniper berries
- pinch of salt

YOU WILL NEED
- A SMALL POUCH OF NATURAL CLOTH

MAKES & KEEPS
Makes 1 charm.
Keeps 1 year.

METHOD
Put the ingredients into the pouch, thinking of your goal.

Squeeze the pouch to release the herbs' fragrance. Hang next to the front door to bring protection to your home and ward off evil.

Good Sleep Charm

Courtesy of Lucy Harmer

INGREDIENTS
- 2 tsp dried mugwort
- 2 tsp dried rue
- 2 tsp dried lavender
- 2 tsp dried angelica
- 2 tsp dried chamomile

YOU WILL NEED
- A SMALL POUCH OF NATURAL CLOTH

MAKES & KEEPS
Makes 1 charm.
Keeps 1 year.

METHOD
Put the ingredients into the pouch, thinking of your goal.

Squeeze the pouch to release the herbs' fragrance. Hang on a bedpost or place under your pillow for protection while asleep and for good dreams.

VARIOUS ODDITIES

Good Luck Charm

Courtesy of Lucy Harmer

INGREDIENTS
- 4 oak leaves
- small piece of dried heather
- 1 tsp dried orange peel
- 1 acorn
- 1 citrine quartz crystal

YOU WILL NEED
- A SMALL POUCH OF NATURAL CLOTH

MAKES & KEEPS
Makes 1 charm.
Keeps 1 year.

METHOD
Put the ingredients into the pouch, thinking of your goal.

Squeeze the pouch to release the herbs' fragrance. Hang it next to the front door or carry it with you through the day.

Prosperous House Charm

Courtesy of Lucy Harmer

INGREDIENTS
- 1 tsp oats
- 1 tsp cloves
- 1 tsp small pieces of cinnamon stick
- 1 tsp mandrake root
- few gold flakes

YOU WILL NEED
- A SMALL POUCH OF NATURAL CLOTH

MAKES & KEEPS
Makes 1 charm.
Keeps 1 year.

METHOD
Put the ingredients into the pouch, thinking of your goal.

Squeeze the pouch to release the herbs' fragrance. Hang it next to the front door to bring abundance and wealth to your home.

Herbal Mouse Deterrent

INGREDIENTS
- 250ml/1 cup water
- 2 tbs basil
- 2 tbs peppermint

Essential oils:
- 2 tsp peppermint
- 2 tsp rosemary
- 2 tsp clove

MAKES & KEEPS
Makes 250ml/1 cup.
Keeps 6 months.

METHOD
Pour boiling water on the herbs and leave to cool. Strain and add the essential oils to the strong herb tea liquid. Mix well.

Soak a cotton wool ball thoroughly in the strong-smelling mix. Place around the mouse's entry point to your home. Repeat every 2–4 weeks.

Stinging Nettle String

INGREDIENTS
- 10 or more fresh nettle stalks (tall, long straight ones are needed)

MAKES & KEEPS
Keeps indefinitely.

METHOD
Wearing gloves, pull the nettle out of the ground. Rub the stinging hairs and strip the leaves off the stem.

Cut approx. 2.5cm/1in off the bottom and top pieces of the stem.

Crush the stem all along with your fingers. Put a fingernail in at the base and open it up all the way along to the top, spreading it open like a book.

Bend the flattened stem over a finger, with the inside facing upwards, to snap the inside fibres. Carefully peel off and discard these.

The nettle's tough outside fibres can be plaited to make a cord. Take 2 or more fibres together and secure one end. Twist both from the other end, then fold them in half. The 2 twisted sides will twist together and naturally form a strong cord.

Leave the cord to dry somewhere warm for 2 hours.

Pungent Pest Control Spray for Plants

Controls pests on outdoor or indoor plants without harming the plant.

INGREDIENTS
- 6 large fresh chillies
- 500ml/2 cups water
- 1 head garlic, peeled and crushed

MAKES & KEEPS
Makes nearly 500ml/2 cups.
Keeps about 1 week in the fridge.

METHOD
Boil the chillies in the water for 15 mins. Add the garlic and leave to steep for several hours or overnight. Strain well through muslin and put in a spray bottle ready to use.

Spray affected plants thoroughly, coating the leaves, stems and earth.

> **Caution**
> Best used outside. Take care when spraying as the chilli can really sting if it gets up your nose or in your eyes. Keep away from children or pets.

Tobacco & Tea Tree Plant Spray

An effective remedy against many insects.

INGREDIENTS
- 500ml/2 cups boiling water
- 1 handful of tobacco (such as a cheap pipe tobacco)
- 100 drops/1 tsp tea tree essential oil

MAKES & KEEPS
Makes nearly 500ml/2 cups.
Keeps about 5 days in the fridge.

METHOD
Pour the boiling water over the tobacco. Leave to cool. Strain and add the tea tree essential oil and put in a spray bottle.

Spray affected plants.

Eco Sudsy Car Soap

A soapy mix that is perfect for washing the car.

INGREDIENTS
- 250ml/1 cup liquid soap
- 4 tbs laundry powder
- 1 large bucket of water

MAKES & KEEPS
Makes 1 wash.

METHOD
Mix the ingredients together as you need them.

Wash the car with the mixture. Rinse well, then use Plant Power Car Wax (right).

Plant Power Car Wax

This lemony wax uses carnauba — a rich, thick wax from the leaves of the carnauba palm from Brazil. You can make this without the carnauba if you can't get it, but it won't be as long-lasting or effective.

INGREDIENTS
- 250ml/1 cup linseed oil
- 4 tbs carnauba wax
- 2 tbs beeswax
- 350ml/1½ cups infused lemon vinegar (p.19)

MAKES & KEEPS
Makes about 750ml/3 cups.
Keeps indefinitely.

METHOD
Heat the ingredients gently (in a double boiler) until the wax has melted. Stir, then pour into a heat-resistant container.

When the mixture is cool, it will solidify. Rub it on the car with a lint-free cloth. Polish to a deep shine with the corner of a cotton duster soaked in vinegar.

Herb Directory

ACHILLEA MILLEFOLIUM
Yarrow

Long used to staunch wounds (on battlefields and elsewhere), yarrow's pinky white flowers and feathery leaves grace many a field and grassland area in temperate zones across the world.

USES Yarrow is used to treat period pains, high blood pressure, blood vessel problems, fevers and respiratory allergies; it can also improve digestion. Although yarrow stops haemorrhaging, taken both internally and used externally, the leaves and flowers are anti-clotting for the circulatory system. Take as tea, tincture, lotion, salve or poultice.

Its root secretions are known to be strengthening to other plants, making them more resistant to disease, and the plant repels harmful insects in the garden.

Some people are allergic to yarrow. Do not use in pregnancy.

AGRIMONIA SSP.
Agrimony

A 1m/3ft tall perennial herb with carrot-like leaves, agrimony is green on top and silvery underneath, with thin spikes of small yellow flowers. It prefers a wet habitat.

USES Agrimony's main quality is its astringency, which means it is drying and toning to mucous membranes. This makes it useful to tone the digestive system, and as a mouthwash for gum disease. It is used to treat bladder and kidney weakness.

Agrimony is also a flower remedy for tension and pressure, especially for those who put on a brave face. Externally it is an excellent healer of wounds, including varicose ulcers. Take as a tea, tincture or external preparation.

AESCULUS HIPPOCASTANUM
Horse Chestnut

This majestic tree, a native of south-eastern Europe, is now cultivated throughout the world. It produces fragrant candles of small flowers and a profusion of brown, shiny, nut-like seeds, protected by spiky green cases.

USES The seeds or 'conkers' are used in internal and external medicines to strengthen blood vessels, especially the veins. In large doses conkers are poisonous — do not mistake it for sweet chestnut and eat too many.

The safe medicinal dose is around 1–2g three times daily. Take as a tincture or in powder form, or apply as a lotion or cream.

ALCHEMILLA VULGARIS
Lady's Mantle

This delicate, yellow-green plant has soft, cape-like leaves that collect dew and tiny, green-yellow flowers. It is usually found in damp meadows, woods and grassy mountains.

USES An excellent general tonic for the womb, lady's mantle stops excess bleeding — menstrual or menopausal — and regulates the female hormonal cycle. The herb also helps women to recover from emotional and physical trauma related to the womb. Being astringent, it can ease diarrhoea and mucous problems of the gut. Its astringency, coupled with an ability to stem bleeding, makes lady's mantle a good healer of wounds. Take as a tea or a tincture, or in a healing salve or poultice. It is not generally used in pregnancy.

HERB DIRECTORY

ALLIUM SATIVUM
Garlic

The bulb of this typical, easy to grow member of the onion family is used in cooking all over the world. Its cousin, *Allium ursinum* (wild garlic), grows all over Europe and can be used similarly.

USES *Garlic is highly effective in fighting infections of all kinds, including coughs and colds, sinusitis and intestinal parasites. Used in treating hayfever and other allergies, it can also lower blood cholesterol and high blood pressure.*

Some research has found it to be a possible neuro-toxin which adversely affects the brain, so it may be best regarded as a medicine for occasional use. Garlic can be eaten raw or made into a powerful tincture, or applied externally to infections.

ALTHAEA OFFICINALIS
Marshmallow

Originally from Africa and now widely cultivated, marsh mallow is a tall perennial herb. It has pale pink flowers and soft, furry, light green leaves.

USES *The leaves and root are used to soften and soothe inflammations of the lungs, guts, urinary tract and skin. The root tends to be used more for guts and lungs, the leaves for the kidneys.*

The root can be chewed by teething babies. In ancient Egypt marsh mallow was mixed with oats and honey to make a sacred sweet offered to the gods.

ALOE VERA
Aloe

This cactus-like plant has long, pointed, succulent leaves edged with small white teeth. It is good to grow as a houseplant, allowing you to split the dark green leaves, reach the clear gel within and use it fresh.

USES *Aloe juice is very rich in vitamins, minerals and health-giving enzymes. It is powerfully detoxifying and an excellent cleanser. Anti-inflammatory for the stomach and colon, aloe juice is used to treat irritable bowel syndrome (IBS) and other digestive inflammations. It helps to heal burns and ulcers and is used in many skin products.*

Do not take in pregnancy or when breast-feeding, or if the kidneys are weak. Do not take internally long-term without regular breaks.

ANGELICA ARCHANGELICA
Angelica

A tall and powerful aromatic bitter of the Umbelliferae family, angelica has tiny flowers with distinctive, umbrella-shaped flower heads. Angelica is found most often growing alongside rivers, preferring damp and shady places. Originally native to Syria, it is now widely cultivated.

Take care when collecting this herb as angelica can easily be mistaken for hemlock, which is poisonous.

USES *Stems and roots can be eaten. In medicinal terms angelica is an aromatic bitter which removes damp and cold from the body. It stimulates the liver and digestive tracts, and is a valuable tonic for the whole system. The root is especially useful for the lungs. All parts of the plant are used, in teas, tinctures and foods. Do not take medicinally during pregnancy.*

ARCTIUM LAPPA
Burdock

In burdock's first year only the leaves appear. They are low to the ground, large and flannelly, with a distinctive smell and feel, being woolly on the underside. In its second year the plant grows a tall, robust stem with leaves and small pinky-purple, thistle-like flowers, which form seed burrs. Native to Europe, it is naturalized in the USA.

USES Burdock is a blood-cleansing herb which is antibiotic, anti-fungal and adaptagenic (protects the body from stress). It lowers blood sugar, stimulates the kidneys, promotes sweating and is used to treat many skin diseases, as well as arthritis and any condition where detoxifying is necessary. The root, leaves and seeds are used in teas, tinctures and foods.

ARMORACIA RUSTICANA
Horseradish

Horseradish is a member of the cabbage family native to Europe and western Asia, then introduced to North America. It has strong, large green leaves and small white flowers.

USES Though best known as a culinary herb, horseradish root is a useful antibiotic and immune-stimulating medicine. It is especially good for infections of the sinuses, lungs, kidneys and guts, and removal of mucus from the body. It is also a strong diuretic that breaks up kidney stones and a stimulant for the circulation.

Horseradish is easy to grow and best used fresh. It is taken internally as a tincture, tea and food, and used externally in lotions.

ARTEMISIA ABSINTHIUM
Wormwood

This bitter herb with small yellow flowers is native to Europe, but now also grown in Asia and the USA. It can easily be grown from seed or by dividing the roots in autumn.

USES Wormwood is used to treat parasite infections of the guts, and as a general tonic. It is a very bitter liver stimulant which affects the central nervous system, and is best used in small amounts. Wormwood was a key ingredient in the liquor 'absinthe', which has mind-altering effects.

Its cousin, A. annua or Chinese wormwood, has been found to be effective against malaria. In countries where the disease is prevalent there have been schemes to encourage growing of Chinese wormwood for use in treatments.

Do not take during pregnancy.

ARTEMISIA VULGARIS
Mugwort

Also known as Chrysanthamum weed, mugwort grows over most of Europe and North America. The under leaves are white, the flowers white/green and small, but in profuse spikes.

USES Mugwort leaves and flower buds can be used to flavour soups, or eaten for their minerals (and their ability to help the body absorb minerals). It is a bitter liver tonic of particular help to the womb, nervous system and stomach.

Mugwort can be taken as a tea or tincture, and can be smoked, like a cigarette, or burned as an incense. It is also used in acupuncture in a procedure called 'moxibustion' where it is burned into the patient's skin. Mugwort is said to help to develop lucid (conscious) dreaming.

Do not take during pregnancy.

HERB DIRECTORY

ASTRAGALUS MEMBRANACEUS
Huang Qi or Milk Vetch

The root of this yellow-flowered member of the vetch family has been used for thousands of years in Chinese medicine for its invigorating qualities. It is native to temperate regions of the Northern Hemisphere.

USES A tonic for the immune system, milk vetch increases our ability to fight off viral disease. It supports the immune system, so helps with chronic fatigue, and also supports people having chemotherapy and radiotherapy. Milk vetch is a general tonic for the digestion, heart and liver, and may also be used to help prolapsed organs, especially the womb. The root is decocted into a tea or made into a tincture.

BAPTISIA TINCTORIA
Wild Indigo

A yellow-flowered perennial in the vetch family, wild indigo is native to North America and widely used in herbal medicine. The name refers to its traditional use as a blue dye.

USES Wild indigo root is used in herbal medicine as an antiseptic blood cleanser and to stimulate immunity against infection. It is especially suited for gut infections including typhus, gastric flu, mouth infections and sepsis anywhere in the body.

AVENA SATIVA
Oatstraw

Oats are a tall grass with straight stems and small seed heads. Herbalists use 'oatstraw' – the green grass and tops of oats before the mature oats are formed – as a powerful medicine. It is native to temperate parts of Europe and Asia, and is widely cultivated around the world.

USES Super-rich in minerals and vitamins, oats are a nutritious, health-enhancing, cholesterol-lowering food.

A tonic and nourishing herb for the nerves, including the brain, oatstraw is used for fatigue, depression and anxiety, and to improve concentration. It can help with insomnia caused by over-exhaustion and may also be used as an aphrodisiac and reproductive tonic. It is taken as a tea or tincture; the grass may be eaten in green smoothies.

BERBERIS VULGARIS
Barberry

Barberry is a thorny deciduous shrub from Africa/Asia and southern Europe, now naturalized in the USA and UK. It has small, leathery leaves, yellow bark and flowers and red berries.

USES In many countries barberry's tart red berries are eaten in savoury dishes and jam. The yellow bark of its stem and root are used as a dye and a powerful medicine.

Barberry contains berberine, an antibacterial, anti-protozoal and anti-parasite antibiotic which is also anti-inflammatory. Used for intestinal infections and eye infections, parasites and malaria, barberry is a bitter stimulant for the liver.

Do not take during pregnancy or long-term (more than 2 months).

MAHONIA AQUIFOLIUM
Oregon Grape

Also known as Mahonia, Oregon grape is an evergreen from North America, grown as an ornamental shrub in the UK and Europe. Growing to 2m/6ft, it has prickly, holly-like leaves, clusters of yellow flowers and small black berries.

USES *A bitter tonic for the liver and digestive system, Oregon grape also contains berberine (so can be used in a similar way to barberry, p.227). It is much used to treat psoriasis, eczema and other skin diseases, being a detoxifier and tonic.*

The inner bark gives a yellow dye, the berries a purple one. Berries can also be eaten, usually cooked and mixed with a sweeter fruit. The root is used in medicines.

Do not take during pregnancy.

CALENDULA OFFICINALIS
Pot Marigold

Originally from southern Europe, pot marigold grows in any temperate climate and is now found all over the world. It is easy to grow and ideal for novice gardeners. The vibrant orange flowers have medicinal use.

USES *Pot marigold is one of the most versatile and amazing plants. The anti-inflammatory flowers heal wounds and work against bacteria, viruses and fungal infections. They are used in preparations for skin problems of all kinds.*

Pot marigold flowers are also effective as a healing remedy for the gut, and for strengthening the liver as well as the nervous system.

BORAGO OFFICINALIS
Borage

Native to the Mediterranean and widely grown elsewhere, borage is a bristly haired, bright green herb with characteristic blue, star-shaped flowers. Star-flower oil is extracted from its seeds. Star-flower oil contains high levels of GLA (Gamma Linoleic Acid) which has many beneficial health effects, including helping to regulate hormone levels, so it can reduce PMS.

USES *Borage is cooling and moistening, and is used in herbal medicine as an adrenal tonic for stress, exhaustion and depression. It soothes stomach inflammations and reduces catarrh in the body.*

Borage leaves and flowers can be eaten and both are delicious. The leaves contain low levels of pyrrolixidine alkaloids, so there are some concerns about borage's safety, as in high doses these damage the liver. Take borage for a few weeks at a time only, and do not take if you have any liver disease or weakness. If in doubt, consult a medical herbalist.

CAPSICUM SPP.
Cayenne Pepper

Cayenne is a hot chilli pepper with long green fruits which usually turn red on ripening. It is native to both South and Central America.

USES *Cayenne pepper fruits are taken as a powerful circulatory stimulant, dilating blood vessels and speeding up flow around the body. The plant speeds up metabolism, helps to burn fat and suppresses the appetite: it is also said to be an aphrodisiac.*

Cayenne pepper is consumed as a powder or tincture, or taken externally as a warming painkiller. It is also used as a spray to deter insects on other plants. Do not use on broken skin or delicate areas, and keep away from the eyes.

Do not take medicinal doses in pregnancy.

HERB DIRECTORY

CHELIDONIUM MAJUS
Greater Celandine

A member of the poppy family with small yellow flowers, the stem of greater celandines gives an orange latex. (Latex is a milky exudate that some plants contain, including opium in poppies and rubber from rubber plants.) Native to Europe, it is widely grown in the USA.

USES A bitter tonic for all manner of liver and gall-bladder diseases, greater celandine is also a mild sedative for the internal organs. It is used to treat whooping cough, asthma and bronchitis with spasm, and for pain in the digestive system. The herb is taken and applied for eczema, and for eye disease and cancers. It is used as a tea, tincture and lotion, and the latex can be directly applied to warts.

Do not take during pregnancy.

CRATAEGUS MONOGYNA
Hawthorn

This wonderful common hedgerow and field tree with its rugged bark, profusion of white-pink flowers and red berries is found throughout Europe. Several North American cousins have similar medicinal properties, including *Crataegus chrysocarpa* (fireberry hawthorn) and *C. douglasii* (black hawthorn) as well as *C. pinnatifida* (Chinese hawthorn).

USES In German herbal medicine hawthorn is known as 'the mother of the heart', and its flowering tops and berries are used to treat all manner of heart disease: angina, abnormal heart rhythms, heart failure, high blood pressure and diseases of the arteries.

CIMICIFUGA RACEMOSA
Black Cohosh

A graceful woodland perennial from the USA, now naturalized in Europe, black cohosh has long, bending spikes of white flowers (1m/3ft in length). Also known as *Actaea racemosa*, black cohosh root was traditionally used for medicine by many Native American tribes.

USES An anti-inflammatory, black cohosh is very helpful for sciatica, back pain, cramp, arthritis and sometimes for migraines. It is a relaxing nerve tonic which can quieten a cough.

Black cohosh can also be helpful for period pains, and for painful breasts and headaches caused by hormonal imbalance, as well as menopausal hot sweats.

Do not use in pregnancy or when breast-feeding. Do not take for more than 6 months without a break.

CURCUMA LONGA
Turmeric

This tropical plant is native to South India, and is widely grown in hot and wet areas of the tropics. Its large green leaves grow to around 1m/3ft and its flowers are whitish green. The yellow rhizomes (roots) are used in cooking. Turmeric is considered to be an exceptionally powerful medicinal plant.

USES A supreme anti-inflammatory, liver activator and antioxidant blood cleanser, turmeric is useful in any inflammatory condition. These include arthritis, skin disorders, asthma, cancers and heart disease. The herb has been shown to be of help in dementia and diabetes. It is normally used in dried powder form as it is imported from India, but if you can get turmeric fresh try eating it grated, or as a juice — it is amazing. It also makes a bold yellow dye.

229

HERB DIRECTORY

DIOSCOREA VILLOSA
Wild Yam

Native to North and Central America, wild yam will grow in subtropical and temperate zone woodlands. It consists of a vine growing from tubers (potato-like roots), which are the part used in medicine.

USES Wild yam is traditionally used as an antispasmodic, especially for gut spasm or colic, and also as an anti-inflammatory for inflamed bowels and arthritic conditions. It is also used to treat women's hormonal imbalances: common in menopausal mixes, the plant is famous for containing diosgenin, from which the first contraceptive pill was developed. It is taken as a tea, tincture and cream.

ELEUTHEROCOCCUS SENTICOSUS
Siberian Ginseng

Native to Russia, China, Korea and Japan, Siberian ginseng is a woody shrub, 3m/10ft in height, with blackish berries and large, dark green leaves with 3–7 lobes.

USES The root is used as a strong adaptogen (meaning that it helps protect the body from the damaging effects of stress) and stimulant. It is often used to boost long-term immunity, including for people with immunosuppression following radiotherapy or chemotherapy. Siberian ginseng is helpful in any stress-related condition, including those caused by hormonal problems such as post-natal depression and menopausal difficulties.

It is best used for short periods of time. For some people it is too stimulating, causing anxiety and panic, especially in high doses. Siberian ginseng is mostly used as a tea and tincture.

ECHINACEA SPP. (E. PURPUREA AND E. ANGUSTIFOLIA)
Purple Coneflower

Native to the USA but now cultivated and known far and wide, this perennial boasts a lovely, large, daisy-type purple flower. The whole plant (root and flowering tops) is used for medicine.

USES Echinacea is an immune stimulant, helping the body to fight infections and cleaning the blood. It is anti-microbial and can be used to treat boils, ulcers, eczema and any infection anywhere in the body. Good-quality echinacea makes the tongue tingle when you taste it or chew it. It is taken as a tincture, tea and pills.

EQUISETUM SPP. (E. ARVENSE AND E. HYEMALE)
Horsetail

This ancient plant with thin, rigid, dry branching stems and leaves resembles a horse's tail. It likes wet, marshy places and grows up to 65cm/2ft in height.

USES Horsetail is rich in silica in a readily absorbable form. A lack of silica can be recognized by weakness of the hair and nails, multiple allergies, chronic bladder inflammation and muscle and joint problems.

Horsetail helps to stop bleeding, especially of the bladder and reproductive organs, and is also used for urinary incontinence.

Take care not to confuse it with E. palustre (marsh horsetail), which is much larger and is toxic.

FILIPENDULA ULMARIA
Meadowsweet

Also known as 'Queen of the Meadow', this lovely herbaceous perennial, with its shower of creamy-white flowers and distinctive smell, is native to Europe and Asia and naturalized in the USA.

USES *Meadowsweet is a useful anti-inflammatory for the stomach and intestines, and for the joints. It relieves and heals stomach ulcers and heartburn and calms an over-active digestion, so can help to stop diarrhoea. The herb also contains salicylic acid (aspirin), so lowers fevers and thins blood.*

GENTIANA LUTEA
Gentian

Gentian grows in the Alps and other mountainous regions. It has oval leaves and star-shaped yellow flowers, and grows to around 130cm/4ft in height. Its bitter roots are collected in the autumn from plants that are over 8 years old, which is when they first begin to flower.

USES *Gentian stimulates the liver and digestion, regulates blood sugar and is a general tonic. It is used usually in small quantities, with a tincture of the root normally being taken at 2–10 drops per dose. Taken directly on the tongue, gentian can help reduce sugar cravings. Avoid if you suffer from acid indigestion or a stomach ulcer.*

GALIUM APARINE
Cleavers, Goosegrass

This creeping plant grows all over Europe, North America and parts of Asia. Cleavers stays close to the ground and climbs over other plants. Its hairy stems are square, its flowers tiny and white, and its fruits resemble little balls.

USES *Cleavers is used to encourage the lymphatic system to detoxify the body. It is taken for any condition in which toxic build-up could be an issue, including conditions of the skin and joints and certain cancers.*

GINKGO BILOBA
Ginkgo

This magnificent and ancient tree, with green, fan-shaped leaves, has been around for about 190 million years. Growing to 30m/100ft, it is native to China and Japan, but now grown all over the world.

USES *The leaves are famous as a brain medicine, stimulating the flow of blood to the brain. Ginkgo is used to treat memory loss and problems of the central nervous system, including dementia, stroke and multiple sclerosis. It has an anti-clotting effect in the blood.*

Ginkgo can also help with asthma, being strongly anti-allergic and anti-inflammatory. It is usually taken in tincture or tablet form, or as powder.

HERB DIRECTORY

GLYCYRRHIZA GLABRA
Liquorice

A woody stemmed member of the pea family, with creamy-white flowers, liquorice is native to southern Europe and Asia. It is now widely cultivated.

USES Liquorice is a famous sweet, full of delicious natural sugars. It is such a useful medicine that it has been called 'the universal herb'.

An adrenal tonic for exhaustion and fatigue, it is anti-inflammatory for the stomach and guts and soothes the lungs and urinary system. Liquorice also heals externally and can help ulcers and eczema (it makes a very black ointment!).

Do not use during pregnancy, or with liver damage or high blood pressure.

INULA HELENIUM
Elecampane

This robust member of the daisy family is native to Europe, but naturalized in the USA. It grows in many places, preferring shady woods and damp pastures. It grows 1–1.5m/3–5ft tall, with yellow flowers and pointed leaves. The root, dug in autumn from plants over 2–3 years old, is used for medicine.

USES Elecampane root is a warming tonic, especially good for the lungs; it treats coughs, catarrh and serious lung disorders of all kinds. Elecampane root is also useful to improve digestion and to treat piles, debility and exhaustion.

Do not take during pregnancy or if breast-feeding.

HYPERICUM PERFORATUM
St John's Wort

This beautiful wayside weed with small yellow flowers is indigenous to Europe, but introduced in temporate zones of the Americas. If you hold the leaves up to the light, you will find little see-through dots: these are oil glands.

USES In addition to its now famous use as an anti-depressant, St John's wort is taken as a tea, capsules or tincture for stress and anxiety, and to treat damage to and diseases of the nerves (including shingles and multiple sclerosis). It supports the immune system and stimulates the liver. The lovely infused oil is anti-inflammatory, anti-viral and wound-healing.

It can cause sensitivity to sunlight and interacts with some drugs, including the oral contraceptive pill. Seek medical advice if you are taking any medication.

IRIS VERSICOLOR
Blue Flag

This beautiful wetland iris, a native of North America, has characteristic purple yellow and whitish flowers much loved by florists. The root is used in herbal medicine throughout the USA and Europe.

USES Used in small doses, the root has the action of stimulating a sluggish liver; it also improves eczema and other skin diseases, encourages the lymphatic system and moves the bowels. Blue flag root is useful for acne, psoriasis and shingles, and can also help people with an under-active thyroid.

Do not take in pregnancy. It can also cause vomiting in large doses.

HERB DIRECTORY

JUGLANS NIGRA
Black Walnut

This beautiful tree is native to the USA but has been widely introduced in Europe. It produces a fruit that falls with its husk, green, in the autumn, and this green fruit, as well as the leaves and flowers, all have medicinal uses.

USES *The nuts are delicious and nutritious. Interestingly they are especially good for the brain — they even look like little brains!*

Black walnut calms inflammation of the bowels and parasite infestation. It also improves digestion and cleans the blood.

Walnut hulls make a brownish-black dye, while the flower makes a remedy to help adjust to periods of change.

Do not use walnut hulls during pregnancy; the flower remedy is fine at this time.

LARREA TRIDENTATA
Creosote Bush

This fragrant evergreen shrub is a familiar sight in the deserts of the south-western USA and north-western Mexico. Growing to 1–3m/3–9ft in height, it has dark green leaves and yellow flowers.

USES *Tea made from creosote leaves was traditionally used for detoxification, and to treat colds and pain from kidney stones.*

Creosote bush is anti-fungal, anti-microbial, anti-viral and anti-inflammatory; it is also astringent and antioxidant. The plant makes a lovely infused oil which heals wounds and soothes inflammations, bruises and skin infections when applied to the skin.

It may be harmful to the liver taken in large doses over a long period, or in susceptible individuals, so do not take it internally unless done under the guidance of a qualified herbalist.

LACTUCA SPP.
Wild Lettuce

The wild cousin of all the cultivated varieties, wild lettuce has small, slightly prickly leaves and yellow flowers. It is much bitterer than cultivated lettuce. Native to Asia and Europe, it is naturalized in the USA.

USES *Remember* The Tale of Peter Rabbit? *He ate too many of Mr McGregor's lettuces and fell asleep ... Wild lettuce has a latex (a white waxy juice that oozes from the fresh stems) which contains an opiate. The latex forms an opiate-like sedative and painkiller used to treat insomnia, hyperactivity, anxiety and pain of various kinds.*

Wild lettuce is taken in herbal medicine as a tea or tincture. In large doses it causes drowsiness.

LAVANDULA ANGUSTIFOLIA AND SPP.
Lavender

This aromatic, purple-flowered perennial prefers dry, well drained soils and lots of sun. It is grown commercially mainly for production of its essential oil, which is antiseptic and anti-inflammatory. Many related species have similar properties. It has been cultivated across Europe, Asia and Africa for thousands of years.

USES *Lavender is used in cooking cakes and puddings, and sometimes for flavouring cheese.*

Medicinally the herb is relaxing and antiseptic. It encourages liver function and is used to treat high blood pressure, exhaustion, anxiety, insomnia, headaches and painful spasms.

The oil is used neat to heal burns and wounds, and is often used in household and personal care products. It is used also as a tea, tincture and aromatic water. Do not take essential oils internally without professional supervision.

HERB DIRECTORY

LEONURUS CARDIACA
Motherwort

Originally from southern Europe and Asia, motherwort long ago spread across the world. This tall, strong perennial of the mint family has hairy, serrated, 3–5-lobed leaves and lilac to pink flowers round the upper parts of the plant.

USES *From the bitter taste, you can tell that motherwort stimulates the liver (as all bitter herbs do). Its names reflect its main medicinal uses — as a herb to strengthen the heart ('lionheart' in Latin) and to treat women's conditions. Motherwort was particularly used to prevent women developing uterine infections after childbirth, and is still widely taken for menopausal difficulties, especially nervous problems. It is an excellent remedy for heart palpitations and weakness, hence its bold Latin name. It is commonly taken as a tea and tincture.*

MATRICARIA CHAMOMILLA
Chamomile

A much-loved member of the daisy family with small yellow and white flowers and a distinctive fragrance. It is native to Europe and Asia. A close relative, *Anthemis nobile* or Roman chamomile, is similarly used.

USES *Known as 'the mother of the gut', chamomile is a relaxing, anti-spasmodic sedative. It is used for all inflammations of the digestive tract, from top to bottom, and also helps insomnia.*

Chamomile is a mild emmenegogue, meaning it can bring on delayed menstruation, and it has been used traditionally as a tea to treat vomiting in pregnancy. (Pregnant women should not use the essential oil.)

Used as a tea, tincture, infused oil or essential oil, chamomile is also soothing for the skin. People allergic to ragwort are sometimes also sensitive to chamomile.

LOBELIA INFLATA
Lobelia

This hairy-stemmed plant has toothed leaves and small, pale purple flowers that are yellowish inside. It is native to the USA.

USES *Lobelia contains strong alkaloids which relax the muscles; it is particularly good for asthma as it will open and relax the respiratory passages. It can be taken internally, and also applied externally, to relieve muscle spasms and cramps.*

If you are giving up smoking, put a drop or two of the tincture directly on your tongue if you need help to reduce cravings.

Treat lobelia with respect as it is very strong — and only available in the UK through qualified medical herbalists. It will make you sick in large amounts, so can be used as an emetic.

MELISSA OFFICINALIS
Lemon Balm

This sweetly lemon-scented hardy perennial is naturalized all over the UK and USA. Similar to mint in appearance, but with bright green leaves and small whitish flowers, it has also been known as 'heart's delight'.

USES *An effective sedative, lemon balm is good for insomnia, headaches, anxiety, stress and hyperactivity. The flowering tops are taken to increase mental stamina, and as a digestive herb.*

As well as bringing a fever down, lemon balm is anti-viral internally and externally. It is good for cold sores and shingles, and the fresh juice applied to cuts and grazes helps them heal.

Lemon balm is an antihistamine and therefore good for allergies (including eczemas). It is safe for all to take.

MENTHA PIPERITA AND SPP.

Peppermint

Peppermint is a herbaceous perennial with square stems and opposite dark green pointy leaves, growing 30–90cm/12–35in. It is very easy to cultivate, spreading by underground roots to form new plants. Mints tend to prefer damp and shady habitats, and are easily recognizable by their distinctive smell and taste.

USES *Rich in an essential oil which gives it many of its properties, mint gives a sensation of cooling when applied to the skin. It stimulates the liver and digestion, so is useful for nausea and vomiting, indigestion and heartburn (and often used to treat IBS).*

Mint acts as a stimulant and gives a feeling of improved concentration. It lowers fever, improves appetite and is a nutritious food. The herb is well used as a tea, oil and tincture.

ORIGANUM VULGARE

Oregano

Oregano and its close cousin, *O. marjorana* (marjoram), are native to the Mediterranean and Asia. Both are small-leaved, highly aromatic members of the mint family, with tiny, pink-purple flowers. They prefer the heat and a well-drained soil, but can be surprisingly hardy when grown.

USES *Oregano and marjoram are well-known culinary herbs that lend a distinctive 'Italian' flavour to dishes. Both are very healthful, nutritious and tasty additions to the diet. They are used in traditional medicine for their antiseptic properties, especially in treating stomach and respiratory infections. They are aromatic bitters, helping the digestion.*

OCIMUM BASILICUM

Basil

Basil is a strongly aromatic member of the mint family, with shiny green leaves and very small white flowers. Native to India, it has been cultivated in southern Europe and across Asia for thousands of years. It is easy to grow on a sunny windowsill.

USES *Basil is a delicious and versatile culinary herb. An anti-viral and anti-microbial plant, it is a superb strengthening tonic for the whole body. It helps the digestion and increases milk flow in nursing mothers. Basil makes a relaxing tonic for the nerves and is good for respiratory ailments.*

Its cousin, O. sanctum or holy basil, is considered in Ayurvedic medicine to be a supreme healing tonic. It is sacred to Vaisnavas, being Krishna's most beloved plant.

PANAX GINSENG & P. QUINQUEFOLIUS

Chinese Ginseng & American Ginseng

Panax ginseng, a perennial plant in the ivy family, has small red berries and a fleshy root. It is found mainly in Korea and China. American ginseng is similar but native to North America; it is also cultivated in China. They are both very prized as medicines.

USES *Ginseng is an 'adaptogen', meaning that it protects the body and mind from the damaging effects of stress. It is beneficial to the immune system and can help with recovery from cancer, especially with problems arising from radiotherapy and chemotherapy. It is traditionally used as an aphrodisiac. Too much can lead to agitation (as with too much caffeine).*

PASSIFLORA INCARNATA
Passion Flower

Also known as maypop, this vine has curly tendrils that hang on as it climbs. It produces gorgeous purple flowers, many varieties of which are cultivated for flowers and fruit. It is native to the USA.

USES *The leaves and flowers have long been used as a general relaxing and calming sedative for insomnia and anxiety, epilepsy and high blood pressure. They are a remedy for twitchy limbs, hyperactivity, pain (in particular nerve pain), and to help manage withdrawal from addictions to alcohol and other drugs.*

Do not take high doses in pregnancy. Passion flower can also cause drowsiness.

PLANTAGO SPP:
Ribwort, Plantain

Both herbs are herbaceous perennials. Ribwort (*Plantago lanceolata*) is named for the characteristic veins running straight up the narrow leaves, stem to tip. *Plantago major*, or plantain, is very similar, but with round leaves instead of long. The flowers of both are brownish bobbles at the end of long, square stems. They are native to Europe and Asia, and naturalized in the USA.

USES *Plantain/ribwort are so nutritious that the whole body feels their benefit when they are eaten. As a medicine they tone and dry the mucous membranes of the body, thus helping the lungs, digestive tract, kidney, bladder and reproductive organs. They help to calm allergies and support the lymphatic system; they are also outstanding wound healers.*

PHYTOLACCA DECANDRA
Poke Root

A US native with red stalks, narrow green leaves, small, greenish-white flowers in spikes and black berries, pokeroot grows up to 3m/ 10ft tall. In large doses it is poisonous, but it is a very useful medicine in small amounts.

USES *Poke root helps the lymphatic system and kills parasites in the gut. It is used for sore and swollen glands, for breast disease and to assist the body to rid itself of cancer.*

The herb is anti-inflammatory when applied externally. A tincture made from the fresh root is used in very small amounts, usually not more than 10ml/2 tsp per week (3–4 drops per dose).

Large doses cause vomiting. Do not use in pregnancy.

POLYGONATUM BIFLORUM
True Solomon's Seal

Native to the USA and China, Solomon's seal is cultivated as a garden plant in Europe for its elegant arched stems, from which hang many small white flowers.

USES *The young shoots and leaves can be boiled like asparagus, and the rhizomes ground to make flour for baking.*

The root is taken and applied externally for arthritis and any musculo-skeletal problem, including injuries. Additionally it is a soothing demulcent (meaning it has a softening action) for the lungs and digestion and an adrenal tonic which supports the heart, liver and kidneys. Solomon's seal is a mild sedative and sometimes helps diabetes and high blood pressure.

The aerial parts, especially the berries, are poisonous.

HERB DIRECTORY

ROSA SPP.
Rose

There are over a hundred species of roses found all over the world. The ones advisable to use for medicine or food include *R. canina*, *R. arkansa*, *R. laevigata*, *R. gallica* var. *centifolia* and *R. rugosa*.

USES *The flowers are edible, as are the fruits; known as 'hips', they are exceptionally rich in vitamin C. The seeds contain an oil which is extracted as an antioxidant and scar-reducing agent. Rose is also known to reduce the effects of ageing when applied to the skin.*

Taken internally, rose is an uplifting herb. Helpful to the stomach and digestion, it is also a liver stimulant and tonic for the womb and kidneys. Some species have anti-cancer activity.

Use the listed wild species for food and medicine, not garden hybrids.

RUBUS IDAEUS
Raspberry

This red-fruited plant with a light green prickly stem and leaves that are green on top and white underneath is native to Europe and Asia, but now widely grown. Its close cousins have similar actions. For example, the US black raspberry is a super antioxidant, which seems to have anti-cancer benefits.

USES *The fruit is a delicious and healthy food, rich in antioxidants. Leaves can be taken as a womb tonic for threatened miscarriage, to prepare for pregnancy or as part of infertility treatment. It is also taken as a tea for the last 2–4 months of pregnancy to prepare for childbirth, and taken after birth to nourish the uterus and increase milk production.*

Raspberry's astringency makes it useful to treat diarrhoea, and as a wash for mouth ulcers and tonsillitis.

ROSMARINUS OFFICINALIS
Rosemary

This aromatic, perennial, woody-stemmed shrub is native to the Mediterranean and needs plenty of sunlight to flourish fully. Its green-white, needle-like leaves and purple/pink/white or blue flowers smell strongly of the essential oil in which rosemary is rich.

USES *Both the fresh and dried herb and the essential oil are often used in medicines, foods and household products as a good anti-bacterial.*

Rosemary promotes the circulation, especially the blood flow to the brain. It is used to treat headaches, depression and weakness, to stimulate the liver and digestion and to strengthen the heart.

Make a tea or tincture of the flowering tops for internal use. Do not take the essential oil internally without some professional supervision.

SALIX ALBA AND SPP.
White Willow

These beautiful trees love damp places, especially river banks. They have flexible wood and green-white leaves, and bees love their small, pollen-rich flowers. The anti-inflammatory drug salicylic acid (aspirin) was first isolated from white willow bark in 1838. Willows grow in most temperate zones of the world.

USES *Willow is also used to fuel ecologically effective and sustainable heating systems, as it grows very fast and takes more CO_2 from the air when it grows than it releases when it is burned. It is a good charcoal-making plant. You can also steam the young leaves and eat them.*

Willow bark is an antiseptic anti-inflammatory and a mild painkiller that reduces fevers. It is used for arthritis, headaches and stomach inflammation. Avoid if you are allergic to aspirin.

HERB DIRECTORY

SAMBUCUS SPP.
Elder

Sambucus nigra in Europe and *S. canadensis* in the USA is a small tree or large shrub. Common in the UK, Europe and North America, it produces creamy white clusters of small flowers which develop into small, juicy, purple-black berries.

USES The flowers and leaves increase sweating, are diuretic and anti-inflammatory. They are used in teas, tinctures and lotions for coughs and colds, and to treat arthritis and rheumatism.

The berries are rich in vitamin C and are a powerful anti-viral agent. They have a normalizing effect on the bowel and so can be used to help diarrhoea, though they are also a mild laxative.

SCUTELLARIA LATERIFLORA
Skullcap

A perennial member of the mint family, this herb loves wet habitats. It has nettle-like leaves with serrated edges and blue-pink flowers. It is native to the USA and is cultivated in Europe.

USES Skullcap is good for the nerves, and is widely used all over the world for almost any problem of the nervous system. It reduces anxiety, helps relaxation and aids recovery from debility caused by long periods of over-activity and over-work. Related species are similarly used.

SCUTELLARIA BAICALENSIS
Baical Skullcap – Huang Qin

A herbaceous perennial from China with purple-blue flowers and lance-shaped leaves, baical skullcap grows to 30–120cm/1–4ft in height. In China it is cultivated both as an ornamental plant and an important medicine. It is now also widely grown in the USA.

USES The yellow root is one of Chinese medicine's fundamental herbs, used 'to clear heat' from the body. An exceptional blood cleanser, it is useful for detoxing and for fighting infections – especially fevers of the lungs, throat, nose and sinuses, when the mucus is thick and yellow.

Baical skullcap stops bleeding and aids the healing of wounds. A liver tonic, it can be used in place of golden seal, which is endangered.

Do not use in pregnancy except under some form of professional supervision.

SALVIA OFFICINALIS AND SPP.
Common Sage

An aromatic flowering herb in the mint family, common sage has grey-green leaves and lilac flowers. It is a Mediterranean native, but is now widely naturalized.

USES Sage is a culinary herb, delicious in savoury dishes and salads.

It is used all over the world as a medicine for infections, lung and digestive disorders and skin problems. It is also an excellent general tonic for weakness and debility following illness.

Sage is a nourishing tonic for the brain and can relieve excessive sweating, including that occurring during menopause. Externally it helps to speed the healing of bruises and inflammations.

Do not take medicinal doses if pregnant (as a spice in food it is fine), or if epileptic.

SILYBUM MARIANUM
Milk Thistle

This robust, pink-purple-flowered thistle is native to Europe. It has prickly, variegated green and white leaves and can grow up to 1.5m/5ft tall. Milk thistle is widely cultivated, and its seeds have been used in healing for over 2000 years.

USES Milk thistle seeds are a very powerful healing agent for the liver, both protecting it from toxins and encouraging its regeneration. The herb is used to treat serious liver problems, including hepatitis and liver damage from drug and alcohol use. Milk thistle can be taken to protect the liver from the toxicity of drugs, including those used in medical treatment, but this can make medications less effective as it speeds up their removal from the body. The ground seeds are commonly taken as capsules or tea.

STACHYS OFFICINALIS
Wood Betony

Also known as *Stachys officinalis*, this perennial herb is native to grasslands in Europe, North Africa and Asia. It has smallish, toothed leaves and clusters of purple flowers, on spikes that grow to 30–60cm/1–2ft tall. It is cultivated in North America and sometimes is found naturalized.

USES Wood betony is a very powerful remedy for the stomach and the nervous system. It is a bitter tonic, especially beneficial for the brain. A tea or tincture is used to treat dizziness and dementia, as well as a sluggish liver, gall-bladder problems and poor digestion.

Do not take during pregnancy.

SOLIDAGO SPP.
Goldenrod

Native to the USA and introduced in Europe, goldenrod is a herbaceous perennial with a lovely spike of pollen-heavy yellow flowers.

USES Goldenrod flowers, seeds and leaves can be added to soups, stews and stir-fries.

It is a good tonic herb for the kidneys, even being used to treat serious problems such as nephritis, and also supports the bladder and prostate.

Goldenrod is an anti-catarrhal and anti-inflammatory tonic to the mucous membranes, used to treat the digestive system and chronic mucus in the nose, throat and ears. It is taken as a tincture or tea.

STELLARIA MEDIA
Chickweed

This creeping annual grows in the colder seasons in many locations in Europe and North America. Its Latin name comes from its tiny, star-shaped white flowers which peep out from its bright green leaves, shaped like mice's ears.

USES Chickweed is very tasty and nutritious, good to eat raw or lightly cooked; it is also great food for chickens. In herbal medicine it is used for skin diseases and arthritis, and for bronchitis and lung disease. The plant is taken internally as a tea or tincture and externally as a cream, ointment or infused oil.

HERB DIRECTORY

SYMPHYTUM OFFICINALE
Comfrey

Comfrey thrives in damp and cool conditions. It has fleshy, dark green, hairy leaves and blue-purple, or sometimes white-pink, flowers. Its black roots conceal a white, gloopy (mucilaginous) interior.

USES Also known as knitbone, comfrey considerably speeds the healing of connective tissue (ligaments, tendons, bones and skin). It is used inside and out as tea and tincture, but the root is not taken internally as it contains pyrrolizidine alkaloids, toxic to the liver in large amounts.

People with liver problems and those taking drugs or medications should avoid comfrey. Otherwise the leaves are fine for short-term use.

Do not use on open wounds as comfrey makes the skin heal so quickly it can heal over dirt or infection, tending to form raised scars.

THUJA OCCIDENTALIS
White Cedar

An evergreen in the cypress family bearing very small cones, white cedar is native to eastern North America and grown in Europe as an ornamental plant. The branches, stem and tiny, flat, scale-like leaves contain a strong essential oil.

USES The plant is traditionally used to treat menstrual problems, headaches and heart ailments.

It is a diuretic used to relieve rheumatism and also helps catarrhal chest complaints. The herb is also used to reduce growths, including warts.

Liquid extracts, tinctures and tea made from white cedar are taken internally in very small doses (the tincture generally used at 5ml/1 tsp a week). The essential oil is used externally.

Do not take when pregnant or breast-feeding.

TARAXACUM OFFICINALE
Dandelion

A common, yellow-flowered weed that grows every year from its deep root. Leaves are long and toothed, growing from a central flower stalk. The cluster of flowers later forms a seed head of hundreds of tiny seeds with fluffy hairs attached, enabling it to travel to new locations on the wind. It is native to Europe, Asia and the Americas.

USES The roots and leaves of dandelion are very nutritious and used as foods and medicines everywhere the herb grows. Medicinally the leaves are a powerful diuretic and kidney and liver tonic. The root is a strong liver tonic and stimulant, and a gentle laxative.

Dandelion is used to detoxify and cleanse the body in treating skin and joint problems, cancers, headaches and general weakness.

THYMUS SPP.
Thyme

There are many species of this small-leaved, aromatic herb with woody stems and tiny pink flowers. *Thyme serpyllum*, or wild thyme, is native to southern Europe and a cultivated variety of this, *T. vulgaris*, is grown all around the world.

USES Thyme contains an essential oil high in 'thymol', a very potent antiseptic. It is used against infections, particularly of the lungs and the guts, including worms. As it is relaxing for spasm, thyme is helpful for asthma and tight, aching muscles. It is a good general tonic.

Do not use the essential oil when pregnant, and never take internally in any but the minutest amounts (and not even these if you have liver or kidney problems).

TRIFOLIUM PRATENSE
Red Clover

A beautiful, low-growing meadow flower with pink, globe-shaped flowerheads made of many tiny flowers. White markings decorate the 3-lobed leaves (occasionally you may find a 4-leaved clover, said to be lucky). It is native to Europe, Asia and Africa and is naturalized in North America.

USES *This is a very nourishing flower to eat any time, including during pregnancy. Red clover was traditionally used for coughs and respiratory problems, and also in treating cancer; it helps to stimulate the immune system into healthy functioning. The herb also has a mildly blood-thinning effect and is helpful for menopausal problems such as hot flushes.*

Do not take red clover if you are on warfarin or other blood thinners.

UMBILICUS RUPESTRIS
Navelwort or Wall Pennywort

Native to Europe, navelwort grows on walls in shady places. It is a fleshy succulent with round leaves. The stem in the middle, which can be found all year round, is more prolific in the summer months when the flower spikes grow.

USES *It is delicious to eat and can be gathered in all seasons. Navelwort juice is cooling and eases pains, both taken internally and applied externally.*

Apply the juice or fresh poultice, or an ointment, to painful ears, painful piles, wounds, gout, nerve pains and sore throats. Take navelwort as a juice or tea for pains in the kidneys and digestive system.

TUSSILAGO FARFARA
Coltsfoot

Coltsfoot is native to Europe, and can now be found in Canada and America's northeastern states. Its yellow dandelion-like flowers emerge in late winter to early spring. They then die down, and a month or so later the heart-shaped grey-green leaves appear.

USES *Both the leaves and flowers of coltsfoot are an excellent expectorant and strengthening lung tonic.*

Like comfrey it contains pyrrolizidine alkaloids, which in large amounts are toxic to the liver. Therefore coltsfoot is not recommended for long periods of use, nor for people with liver problems or those taking drugs or medications (because most of these are toxic to the liver).

Do not take while pregnant or breast-feeding.

URTICA DIOICA
Stinging Nettle

This perennial plant can grow over 1m/3ft tall from its network of thin whitish roots, and has green, sharply serrated leaves. The undersides of the leaves are covered in fine, histamine-containing hairs which sting you if touched. It is native to Europe, USA, Asia and North Africa.

USES *Nettles are one of the great panaceas of the plant world. Rich in minerals and vitamins and amino acids, they are one of the best, and easiest to find, wild plants to use as a food. The new green tops and the seeds are edible. Nettle leaves are used for arthritis, skin problems and allergies, and are generally detoxifying and cleansing. Nettle root helps the prostate gland.*

HERB DIRECTORY

VACCINIUM
Bilberry or Huckleberry

Bilberry is a low-growing, shrubby member of the heather family which grows on heaths, moors and mountainous areas of Europe, Asia and America. It has small leaves and produces many small, deep red-black fruits (resembling small blueberries).

USES Bilberries are edible. The leaves and berries gathered before the berries ripen are used to protect the eyesight and help with macular degeneration, cataracts and diabetic eye problems. Bilberries can also help with high blood sugar, so are ideal for diabetics.

Like other deep red/black fruits, the plant nourishes and helps to repair arteries and the veins. Fresh berries are laxative, but dried ones are anti-infective and binding, so good for diarrhoea. Leaves are also used to treat cystitis, kidney and bladder complaints.

VERBASCUM THAPSUS
Mullein

Native to Europe but naturalized in the USA, this beautiful herb has a tall spike of yellow flowers at its top and pale green/grey leaves. They feel as soft as velvet, being densely covered with fine hairs.

USES Mullein is so rich in vitamins and minerals that it is a good herb to drink as tea regularly — though not very nice to eat because of its furriness!

Mullein leaves and flowers soothe and calm inflamed lungs, helping deep and painful coughing, and ease the expectoration of mucus. They are also useful in treating hayfever and bed-wetting. Externally mullein is a good wound healer and helps to reduce piles. An oil made from the flowers is specific for earache.

It is used in smoking mixtures.

VALERIANA OFFICINALIS
Valerian

Every spring this perennial begins to grow from a bundle of rhizome and thin roots to a tall, leafy plant, with flowerheads of many small, pale, white and pinkish flowers. It prefers damp soil. It is native to Europe and northern Asia, but is much used in herbal medicine in the USA.

USES The part of valerian used in medicine is the root and rhizome, and they have an extraordinary smell — you either love or hate it! Valerian is one of the most researched herbal sedatives and is used for anxiety, stress, insomnia and physical tension. It is taken as a tea, tablets and tincture. Cats (including lions) adore it.

Valerian can cause drowsiness and may react with sedative drugs.

VERBENA SPP.
Vervain

Vervain flowers form spikes of small, blue-purple blossoms. The European plant *V. officinalis* is spindly with purplish flowers, and its US cousin, *V. hastate*, has sturdier stems and blue flowers. Both plants are used in similar ways.

USES Vervain is a key herb for treating the nervous system. Herbalists value the plant as a relaxing nervine used for stress, tension and nervous exhaustion. It is also a stimulating bitter tonic for the liver.

Vervain was one of the most important plants of the Druids, being considered a powerful magical plant.

Do not use during pregnancy.

VIBURNUM OPULUS
Guelder Rose/Cramp Bark

This deciduous shrub, almost a tree, has vine-like leaves, white flowers and red berries. It is native to the USA and Europe. An American cousin, *Viburnum prunifolium* (black haw), is also used in herbal medicine.

USES As the name cramp bark suggests, this plant is a muscle-relaxant and anti-spasmodic. Cramp bark is used to treat muscle cramps and tension, period pains and threatened abortion (it relaxes the womb), asthma (it relaxes spasm in the bronchial tubes of the lungs), colic and spastic pains in the gut. The herb also improves the circulation by opening blood vessels. Its American relative, black haw, is used similarly; it also treats morning sickness and problems in menopause.

VITEX AGNUS-CASTUS
Chasteberry

The tiny, yellow-red berries of this beautiful, aromatic Mediterranean flowering tree are known as 'monkspepper' after its 'an-aphrodisiac' effect.

USES Chasteberry is used to treat pre-menstrual syndrome and menstrual irregularities, including those associated with menopause and polycystic ovarian syndrome. The plant can also help some women to conceive if infertility is caused by low progesterone levels, and it increases production of breast milk. Chasteberry can also be useful for acne and headaches associated with hormone imbalance, and can calm acne in teenage boys.

VIOLA SPP.
Sweet Violet & Heartsease (Johnny-Jump-Up)

These two members of the violet family (*Viola odorata* and *V. tricolor*) are native to Europe and naturalized in the USA. Sweet violets have a delicious smell and are the traditional violet colour. Heartsease is a 'tricolor' pansy, with white, purple and yellow flowers.

USES Both herbs are used to treat bronchitis, asthma and other lung problems. They are also useful for cystitis and an irritated bladder.

Sweet violet helps to relieve congested lymph flow. It has also been used, internally and externally, in treating cancers and growths, both as a curative and a pain reliever.

Heartsease is particularly used for wet eczema and other skin diseases with sticky discharges.

ZINGIBER OFFICINALE
Ginger

Ginger is widely known as a pungent culinary spice. The root of this relative of turmeric and cardamom originated in Asia, but is now used all over the world. It is a perennial plant resembling a reed, with lovely yellow flowers.

USES Used in cooking savoury and sweet dishes, as well as in pickles and sweets, ginger stimulates the whole system. The herb makes you sweat and so reduces fever, clears mucus from the head, sinuses and lungs, and relaxes and stimulates the digestion, thus helping to treat indigestion, wind and colic. Ginger helps to reduce nausea of all kinds, and is safe to take for morning sickness in pregnancy.

It is also an excellent circulatory stimulant and can help to reduce high blood pressure.

CONTRIBUTORS

I offer grateful thanks to the following plant experts who have kindly shared their recipes.

Louise Berliner is an artist and writer from Massachusetts, USA, who loves to play with herbs.
See pp.*123, 154*

ChaNan Bonser practises creative kinesiology and runs 'Elemental Medicine', offering physiotherapy treatments in Wales, UK.
See pp.*66, 174, 179*

Lynn-Amanda Brown is a multi-faceted therapist and healer who works in alliance with the sacred energies of the natural world. She lives in Wales, UK.
See p.*173*

Stephen Buhner is the award-winning author of 15 books on nature, indigenous cultures, the environment and herbal medicine. He is one of the co-founders of The Foundation for Gaian Studies, an organization that explores and promotes our reconnection with Nature. He lives in New Mexico, USA.
See pp.*120, 170*

Anne Chiotis is a herbalist based in Wolverhampton, UK.
See p.*80*

Sharon Cohen is a native plant expert living in the forests of Maryland, USA. She runs Native Design, a company providing heart-based ecological restoration and garden design.
See p.*141*

Michael Cole is a UK forager passionate about making Leafu – a protein-rich food made from nettles and other edible wild greens.
See p.*57*

Rachel Corby is a gardener, forager and writer based in Stroud, UK. She runs Gateways to Eden, offering treatments and running workshops on the power of plants.
See pp.*53, 163*

Eliot Cowan developed Plant Spirit Medicine and lives at the Blue Deer Center, New York State, USA. He travels widely, teaching, healing and promoting a balanced relationship with the human and other-than-human worlds.
See pp.*85, 86*

Lesley Cunningham knows a lot about treating her horse friends with herbs.
See pp.*138, 139*

Anna Dowding is a true domestic alchemist from North Wales, UK, who invents brilliant lotions and potions and co-runs Getafix first aid and wild water sports experiences.
See p.*131*

Geoff Edwards was a herbalist for many years and now runs UK-based Ta'i chi centre Wutan Bournemouth.
See p.*99*

Teri Evans is a medical herbalist and runs Cunnynge Herbs in Shropshire, UK. Here she sells artisan herbal tinctures and holds workshops on using herbs.
See pp.*27, 33, 38, 64, 76, 88, 130, 178, 179, 180, 181, 182, 184, 185, 187, 189, 190, 191, 192, 201, 202, 203, 205, 207, 209, 210, 211, 214*

Annie Gardner is a herbalist based in Totnes, UK.
See p.*152*

Monika Ghent is a herbalist and a Plant Spirit Medicine Healer. She runs Dreaming Willow natural therapies in Toronto, Canada, and designs and makes natural skin care products.
See pp.*77, 132, 183, 184, 188, 190, 192, 193, 209, 212*

Lucy Harmer is an international author and teacher based in Geneva, Switzerland. She is also a feng shui and space clearing expert, and a

CONTRIBUTORS

high priestess on the Celtic Shamanic Path.
See pp.*36, 59, 186, 217, 218, 219*

Shelley Harrison is a healer and yoga teacher based near Ottawa, Canada.
See p.*152*

Christine Herren-Valette is a Swiss herbalist who trained as a medical nurse. She now runs a successful small business, Sancta Herba, making herbal products.
See pp.*63, 114, 175, 193*

Johanna Herzog is a herbalist and Plant Spirit Medicine practitioner. She runs a school of medicinal plants, or Heilkraeuterausbildung, near Hamburg, Germany.
See pp.*64, 74, 191, 208*

Wizz Holland is a Plant Spirit Medicine healer, forager, fire keeper and animal communicator. Also a poet and artist, she is based in Devon, UK.
See pp.*55, 56, 145*

Louise Idoux is a medical herbalist from Shropshire, UK. She runs the Oswestry Herbarium, providing treatments and courses on making herbal products.
See pp.*61, 78, 96, 102, 136*

Catherine Johnson is a consulting medical herbalist in Wales, UK.
See pp.*89, 122*

Barbara Jones is an experienced veterinary surgeon who runs Vet Holistic in Shropshire, UK.
See pp.*135, 136, 137, 138*

Steve Kippax is a herbalist and TCM practitioner. He is Head of Complementary Medicine at The Third Space Medicine, London's leading integrated medical centre.
See pp.*96, 102*

Dedj Leibbrandt is a herbalist and teacher in Hampshire, UK. Dedj was awarded a Fellowship of the National Institute of Medical Herbalists for her work on acute medicine and herbal first aid.
See pp.*70, 82, 91, 101, 103, 106, 111, 121, 122, 135, 139*

Marc Luyckx is a domestic alchemist in Switzerland.
See p.*48*

Anne McIntyre is an experienced herbalist, plant grower, writer and teacher, based in the Cotswolds, UK.
See pp.*107, 110, 114, 126, 127, 128, 129, 140, 153, 177*

Neil McNulty is a herbalist, iridologist and facilitator who lives in Zagreb, Croatia. His practice is called Herba Vitalis, and his healing sanctuary is called 'Wild at Heart'.
See p.*62*

Alaina Mecklenburgh is a master herbalist practising in the southern part of the Lake District in the UK.
See p.*213*

Joe Nasr is a medical herbalist, osteopath and senior lecturer in herbal medicine, as well as a dedicated and experienced plant distiller. In 1997 Joe founded Avicenna, a company producing unique, high-quality herbal products in Wales, UK.
See pp.*65, 133*

Jenny Pao is a holistic health practitioner and aromatherapist. She runs Nectar Essences, a company based in San Francisco, USA.
See pp.*180*

Annie Powell runs the Little Green Cream Company, a small ethical company making top-quality skincare products in Wales, UK.
See pp.*66, 171, 177*

Lynn Rawlinson is a consulting medical herbalist and holistic therapist. She lives and works in Merseyside, UK.
See pp.*53, 118, 120, 181, 201, 202*

CONTRIBUTORS

Anna Richardson runs wild food foraging courses for Circle of Life Rediscovery, UK, and is a Forest School leader and author.
See pp.*140, 141*

Melissa Ronaldson is a UK-based herbalist with a passion for snuff. She is co-founder of the Herbal Snuff Company.
See p.*124*

Jeanne Rose is an aromatherapist in San Francisco, USA. She runs 'The Aromatic Plant Project' and is the director and principal tutor of the Institute of Aromatic Studies.
See p.*57*

Anthony Seifert is a Californian herbalist who is on the faculty at the Ohlone Center for Herbal Studies in Berkeley, CA. He works with both humans and animals, and also runs a herbal supply company, Great Blue Heron Botanical Medicine Making Project.
See p.*114*

Sensory Solutions is a UK-based company run by traditional herbalists Karen Lawton and Fiona Heckels. They teach, grow and collect plants to produce beautiful, high-quality remedies.
See pp.*75, 108, 164, 165*

Maida Silverman is an expert on wild plants that grow in New York City, USA, where she has lived all her life.
See p.*179*

Tanya Smart runs the Yemoya company in Glastonbury, Somerset, UK, which makes the best organic soaps ever.
See pp.*196, 198*

Karen Stephenson has created and runs Edible Wild Foods, a wonderful website about foraging and eating wild food. She lives in Ontario, Canada.

See pp.*121, 143, 146, 149, 154, 155, 156, 157, 158, 160, 163, 164, 165, 203*

Iain Stewart is a herbalist working with the Rhizome Community Clinic in Bristol, UK.
See p.*80*

Sucandra devi dasi is a domestic alchemist from Hertfordshire, UK.
See p.*144*

Kamala Todd is an artist based in Malvern, UK, who makes rose petal bead jewellery.
See p.*215*

Michael Vertolli is a Western traditional herbalist who lives in Ontario, Canada. He is the founder and director of the Living Earth School of Herbalism.
See pp.*26, 92*

Emma Warrener is a herbalist in Lincolnshire, UK. She runs Herbs for Health and Wellbeing.
See pp.*195, 206*

Susun Weed is a herbalist and teacher based in Woodstock, USA. She is the voice of the Wise Woman Way.
See pp.*48, 149, 170*

Lucy Wells is a plant spirit medicine practitioner and fire keeper based in Shropshire, UK.
See pp.*57, 76*

Neil Williams is a herbalist who practises in the north-west of England, UK.
See pp.*98, 120*

Sue Wine is a McTimoney chiropractic based in Chester, Cheshire, UK.
See pp.*63, 87, 150*

Mathew Wood is a professional member of the American Herbalist's Guild and the author of six books on herbal medicine. He lives in Oregon, USA.
See pp.*18-19, 116, 117*

SOURCES & FURTHER READING

Books

Bartram, Thomas, 1995. *The Encyclopedia of Herbal Medicine* (Dorset: Grace Publishers)

Bond, Annie B., 2005. *Home Enlightenment* (Kindle edition)

Buhner, Stephen Harrod, 2004. *The Secret Teachings of Plants* (Vermont: Bear & Company)

Buhner, Stephen Harrod, 2002. *The Lost Language of Plants* (Vermont: Chelsea Green Publishing)

Buhner, Stephen Harrod, 1998. *Sacred and Herbal Healing Beers* (Boulder: Siris Books)

Chevallier, Andrew, 1996–2000. *Encyclopedia of Herbal Medicine* (London: Dorling Kindersley)

Corby, Rachel and Studd, Stephen, 2009. *The Medicine Garden* (Preston: The Good Life Press)

Cowan, Eliot, 2014. *Plant Spirit Medicine* (Boulder: Sounds True)

Dau Dayal das, 2014. *The Beautiful Song of God – Srimad Bhagavad Gita* (Llangollen: The Dreaming Butterfly)

Hawes, Zoe, 2010. *Wild Drugs: A Forager's Guide to Healing Plants* (London: Gaia)

Hedley, Christopher and Shaw, Non, 1996. *Non Herbal Remedies: A Practical Beginner's Guide to Making Effective Remedies in the Kitchen* (Bristol: Parragon)

Hoffman, David, 1990. *Holistic Herbal: A Safe and Practical Guide to Making and Using Remedies* (Shaftesbury: HarperCollins)

Hughes, Nathaniel and Owen, Fiona, 2014. *Intuitive Herbalism* (Stroud: Quintessence)

Jeffery, Josie, 2011. *Seedbombs – Going Wild With Flowers* (Lewes: Leaping Hare Press)

McIntyre, Anne, 2011. *Drugs in Pots* (London: Gaia)

Michael, Pamela, 1986. *A Country Harvest* (London: Peerage Books)

Silverman, Maida, 1997. *A City Herbal* (Woodstock: Ash Tree Publishing)

Waller, Pip, 2009. *Holistic Anatomy – An Integrative Guide to the Human Body* (Berkeley: North Atlantic Books)

Weisse, Vivien, 2002. *The Gourmet Weed Cookery Book* (Norderstedt: VIWO)

Wood, Matthew, 1997. *The Book of Herbal Wisdom* (Berkeley: North Atlantic Books)

Yasodananda das, 2013. *Kitchen of Love* (Haarlem: Bhaktimedia.org)

Useful Websites

www.pipwaller.co.uk (my professional website)

www.thedomesticalchemist.com.org (for herbal news and my latest recipes)

www.americanherbalistsguild.com (for finding a herbalist in the USA)

www.anamed.net (for growing *Artemisia annua* in the Tropics)

www.associationofmasterherbalists.co.uk (for finding a herbalist in the UK)

www.ediblewildfood.com (for great foraging information and recipes)

www.gaianstudies.org (for USA-based training from The Foundation for Gaian Studies)

www.globalhealingcenter.com (for information about growing plants in the USA)

www.herbnet.com (for everything herbal in the USA)

www.herbworld.com (for an online encyclopedia with herbal information)

www.mercola.com (for a health information and research site in the USA)

www.nimh.org.uk (the National Institute of Medical Herbalists: for finding a UK herbalist)

www.wddty.com (What Doctors Don't Tell You: A site with interesting reviews of research)

INDEX

A

acid indigestion 101, 231
acne 118, 120, 181, 232, 243
Acne Spot Ointment 120
Acorn Biscuits 141
Acorn Flour 140
acupuncture 226
adaptogens 226, 230, 235
adrenal tonics 232, 236
After-dinner Mouth Freshener 159
aftershave 213
agrimony 76, 116, 224
Agrimony Teachers' Gargle 76
Air-con Shield 91
alcohol 18, 78
All-natural Hot Oil Hair Treatment 207
All-purpose Cleaning Spray 26
allergies 57, 131, 224, 225, 230, 231, 234, 236, 237, 241
aloe 58, 83, 225
Aloe Vera Instant Burn Remedy 83
Aloe Vera Nourish-all 58
American ginseng 235
angelica 155, 175, 225
Angelica Archangel After-dinner Liqueur 175
Angelica Supreme 155
Animal Eardrops 135
Anti-ageing Day Cream 182
Anti-ageing Skin Scrub 201
Anti-allergy Ice Pops 131
Anti-anxiety Drops with Valerian & Rose 115
Anti-bacterial Multi-surface Cleaner 27
Anti-cellulite Body Scrub 185
anti-clotting agents 224, 231
Anti-cold Sore Lip Balm 192
Anti-flu Soup 150
Anti-fungal Ointment 118
Anti-haemorrhage Mix 112
anti-inflammatories 69, 73, 225, 227, 228, 229, 230, 231, 232, 233, 236, 237, 238

Anti-malaria Mix 93
Anti-nausea Suppositories 101
Anti-nausea Tea 100
Anti-psoriasis Laundry Liquid 43
Anti-septic Body Butter 188
Anti-spasmodic Drops 103
Anti-stress Tea 70
anti-viral action 66, 83, 134, 228, 232, 233, 234, 235, 238
Anti-viral Elder 66
Anti-wart Tincture 121
Antibacterial Fabric Softener 49
Antibacterial Honey 79
Antibacterial Laminate & Wooden Floor Cleaner 35
Antibacterial Liquid Handwash 200
Antioxidant Rich Sunscreen 132
Antiseptic Hand Sanitizer 91
Antiseptic Handcream 189
Antiseptic Healing Lotion 83
Antiseptic Mist 78
anxiety 90, 114, 115, 227, 230, 232, 233, 234, 236, 238, 242
Aphrodisiac Brandy 172
aphrodisiacs 172, 227, 228, 235
appetite suppression 60, 228
Apple Cider Vinegar 165
aromatic waters 15, 133–4
arthritis 7, 67, 116, 226, 229, 230, 236, 237, 238, 239, 241
    pets 137
Ashwagandha Night Cap 177
asthma 229, 231, 234, 240, 243
athlete's foot 86, 131

B

Baby Bubbles 197
baby oil 129
Baby Powder for a Dry Bottom 131
Baby-soft Washing Powder 46
baby wipes 131
Baby's First Herbal Tea 126
backs 117, 229
baical skullcap 238
Balancing Tincture for the
    Menopause 114
Balsamic Vinegar 164
barberry 227
Barrier Bar for Busy Hands 66
basil 28, 87, 235
Basil Snifterchief 87
bath bomb 185
bath salts 186
'Beach Hair' Styling Spray for Curls 191
beads 215
Bed Sore Preventative Rub 69
bed-wetting 125, 242
Beech Nut Flapjacks 142
beers 169, 170
Beetroot Lippy 193
Bentonite Clay Cleanser 105
Big Cleanser Smoothie 62
bilberry 159, 242
Birch Aromatic Syrup for Coughs & Sore Throats 64
Birch Massage Oil 74
biscuits 141
Biting Insect Repellent 92
black cohosh 229
black walnut 233
Blackberry & Blackcurrant Brandy 173
bladder 106, 107, 166, 224, 225, 230, 232, 236, 239, 242, 243
bleeding 112, 224, 230, 238
blinis 144
blood cleansing 123, 226, 227, 229, 230, 233, 238
Blood-cleansing Formula 123
blood sugar 226, 231, 242
Blood Thinning Mix for Long-haul Travellers 90
blue flag 232
Blue-Purple Ink 214
body butters 187, 188
boot polish 215
borage 145, 228
borax 43
Bowel Cleanse 104

248

bowels 61, 102, 104, 105, 225, 230, 232, 233, 238
  see also diarrhoea
brain 68, 69, 225, 227, 231, 233, 237, 238, 239
Brain-booster 68
brandy 172, 173, 174
breast cancer 122, 123, 236
breast-feeding 139
Breathe-easy Pot pourri 39
Bright Eyes Wash 97
broken bones 84, 240
bronchial conditions 53, 229, 239, 243
Brown Ink 214
bruises 84, 85, 233, 238
Buckwheat Blinis 144
Bug-busting Mix for Holiday Tums 92
Bug-busting Surface Cleaner 27
Bug Off! Insect-repellent Soap 196
burdock 154, 155, 168, 204, 226
Burdock Anti-dandruff Shampoo 204
burns 83, 225, 233
Buttered Burdock Stems 155
buying herbs 13

C

Calcium-rich Herb Salad 153
calcium tonic 57
calendula see marigold
Calling All Angels Spray 37
Calm & Relaxation Spray 37
Calming Herbal Baths 129
Cancer Treatment Survival Drink 122
cancers 122, 123, 164, 229, 231, 235, 236, 237, 240, 241, 243
carpet cleaner 35
cars 221
Cartilage Healing Salve 117
catarrh 53, 101, 228, 232, 239, 240
catnip 135
Cattail Rice Recipe 154
cayenne pepper 156, 228
Cedar & Southernwood Moth Repellent 50

cellulite 185, 192
cellulitis 74
Chai Tea with Redbush 166
chamomile 26, 79, 134, 234
Chamomile & Marjoram Surface Cleaner 26
change 59, 63, 216, 233
charms 218–19
chasteberry 243
Cheering Tea 70
chemotherapy 122, 227, 230, 235
chickweed 153, 239
Chickweed Sag Paneer 153
Chilblain Oil 63
childbirth 112, 234, 237
Children's Cough Honey 126
Chinese ginseng 235
Choca-coco Sugar Body Scrub 184
chocolate 108, 109, 156, 178, 184, 192
Chocolate Bomb Lip Therapy 192
cholesterol 225, 227
Chronic Diarrhoea Medicine for Pets 136
Cinnamint Toothpaste 209
circulation 75, 87, 95, 134, 144, 174, 224, 226, 228, 237, 242, 243
Citrus Carpet Cleaner 35
Citrus Fresh Deodorant 211
Citrus Hair Spray 191
Citrus Laundry Liquid 42
Citrus, Oat and Honey Soap 195
Clay Soap Alternative 201
Clear Vision Drops 75
cleavers 164, 231
Cleavers Vinegar 164
Cleopatra's Cleanser 178
Coconut Inflammation Beater 69
Coconut Liver Blast 105
Coconut Scrub for Blemishes 202
Cold & Flu Tea 87
Cold Sore Lotion 121
Cold Sore Ointment 118
cold sores 118, 121, 192, 234
colds 53, 63, 87, 97, 165, 225, 233
colic 133, 230, 243
coltsfoot 97, 100, 241
Coltsfoot Expectorant Honey 97

comfrey 8, 80, 82, 84, 145, 203, 240
Comfrey & Elder Shampoo for Dry Hair 203
Comfrey Cream for Speedy Healing 82
Comfrey Fritters 145
Comfrey Oil 80
compresses 19
Computer Energy Booster Spray 36
Concentrated Lavender Laundry Liquid 42
Contractions Booster 112
cookies 141, 143
Cornflower & Rosemary Dry Shampoo 204
cornsilk 63
Cough Tea 126
coughs 64, 65, 76, 80, 97, 99, 100, 101, 125, 126, 177, 225, 229, 232, 241, 242
crackers 149
cramp 229, 234, 243
  see also spasm
cramp bark 243
Cramp-relieving Tincture 114
Cream for Vaginal Thrush 110
creams 20–1
creosote bush 233
Crystallized Ginger 162
cystitis 106, 166, 242, 243
Cystitis Regime 106
Cystitis Tea 106

D

daisy 84, 85
Daisy Bruise Ointment 85
dandelion 168, 171, 240
Dandelion & Burdock 168
Dandelion Champagne 171
Dandelion Coffee 171
dandruff 204
decoctions 15
Deep Sleep Spray 37
dehydration 88, 93, 127
  see also rehydration
dementia 229, 231, 239
deodorant 210–12

249

depression 116, 164, 227, 228, 230, 232, 237
Desert-style Moth Repellent 50
Detox Complex 61
Detox Tea 61
detoxification 57, 61, 63, 104, 225, 226, 228, 231, 233, 238, 240, 241
Detoxing Mineral Vinegar 57
devil's claw 137
diabetes 229, 236, 242
diarrhoea 93, 127, 224, 231, 237, 238, 242
 pets 136
Diarrhoea Stopper 93
digestion 102, 126, 140, 143, 175, 224, 225, 227, 228, 229, 231, 232, 233, 234, 235, 236, 237, 238, 239, 241, 243
 see also gut; indigestion; stomach
diosgenin 230
disinfectants 29, 31
diuretics 96, 164, 226, 238, 240
dizziness 114, 239
Dogs' Arthritis Medicine 137
Dogs' Upset Stomach Powder 136
Doux-Baiser Lipstick 193
drain cleaner 32
Drawing Ointment 120
Dry-bed Syrup 125
drying herbs 13, 16
dyes 227, 228, 229, 233

E

Ear Oil 77
ears 77, 79, 239, 241
earache 76, 77, 86, 242
 pets 135
Easy Cherry Syrup 166
Easy Iron Tonic 56
echinacea 65, 230
Eco-powered Laundry Whitener 47
Eco-powered Oven Cleaner with Basil 28
Eco Sudsy Car Soap 221
eczema 118, 126, 164, 228, 229, 230, 232, 234, 243
elder 55, 66, 67, 145, 159, 162, 171, 177, 203, 238
Elder, Rosehip & Rowanberry Oxymel 55
Elderberry Oxymel 67
Elderflower Champagne 171
Elderflower Cordial 162
Elderflower Fritters 145
Elderflower Wine 177
Elders' Alcohol-Free Tonic 68
Elders' Sherry Tonic 67
elecampane 161, 232
Elecampane Sweets 161
Emotional Balancing Spray 37
epilepsy 236
Equinox Tea for the Changing Seasons 63
equipment 16–17, 23
essential oils 21, 22, 39, 195, 204
Exfoliating Seaweed Scrub 185
exhaustion 227, 228, 232, 233, 242
eyes 75, 79, 97, 183, 227, 229, 242
 pets 137

F

fabric conditioners 48–9
face masks/packs 178, 179
Facial Serum for Sun-damaged Skin 183
False Solomon's Seal & Teasel for Joints 116
fat burning 60, 69, 228
fatigue 227, 232
feet 86, 131, 191
Fennel Oatcakes 148
fertility 108, 115, 237, 243
fever 88, 165, 175, 224, 231, 234, 235, 238, 243
Fiery Muscle Rub 74
Findhorn 12
Fire Cider 165
Fissure Salve 120
flapjacks 142
flatulence *see* wind
Flaxseed Rehydration Tea 52
fleas 44, 92, 136
floor cleaners 30, 35
flu 87, 150, 227
fluid extracts 18

Fly Repellant 38
flying 90, 91
Foot & Leg Spray 191
Forest & Corn Goddess Cookies 141
Forsythia Syrup 157
Friar's Balsam 98
fritters 145
fruit leathers 56
Fruity Body Custard 187
fungal infections 86, 118, 122, 131, 181, 226, 228, 233
 horses 138
Fungal Toe Nail Cure 122
furniture polishes 32–4

G

gall bladder 229, 239
Gardeners' Soap for Dirty Nails 197
gargles 76, 97, 128, 165, 210
garlic 65, 139, 151, 152, 225
Garlic & Echinacea Infection-busting Tincture 65
gentian 231
Gentle Rose Toner for Mature Skin 180
Gentle Soapnut Laundry Liquid 44
ginger 63, 160, 162, 169, 243
ginger beer 169
Ginger Pop 169
ginkgo 231
ginseng 59, 67, 230, 235
glass cleaner 30
Gobo – Burdock Roots Japanese-style 154
goldenrod 163, 239
Goldenrod Vinegar 164
Good Luck Charm 219
Good Sleep Charm 218
goose grass *see* cleavers
Gorse Liqueur 174
Gorse Wine 177
gout 241
graze remedy 78
greater celandine 229
Green Dragon Shaving Oil 213
grief 71, 116, 165
Grief Tea 71
Gripe Water 133

growing herbs 12
gum disease 210, 224
gut 165, 224, 225, 226, 227, 228, 230, 231, 232, 234, 236, 240, 243

H

haemorrhoids *see* piles
hair 134, 165, 191, 196, 202-8, 230
Hair Growth Tonic 208
Hair Mud 205
hands 66, 91, 130, 182, 189, 190, 200, 201
   see also nails
hangover cure 88
Happy Home Charm 218
Happy House Air Spray 36
hawthorn 96, 99, 157, 158, 229
Hawthorn Flower Syrup 157
hayfever 89, 131, 177, 225, 242
Hayfever Mead 89
head lice 132, 206
Headache Powders 88
headaches 88, 89, 114, 229, 233, 234, 237, 240, 243
Heal-all Marigold Cream 81
Heal-all Marigold Oil 81
Healing Skin Scrub 202
heart 75, 96, 227, 229, 234, 236, 237, 240
Heart & Blood Pressure Tea 96
heartburn 102, 133, 231, 235
Heartburn Tea 102
heartsease 243
henbane 103
Herb Pesto 152
Herb Salt 147
Herbal Anti-depressant 116
Herbal Aspirin 88
Herbal House Cleansing Smudge Stick 217
Herbal 'HRT' Cream 113
Herbal Mouse Deterrent 219
Herbal Tonic for Prostate Health 115
Herbie Aftershave 213
herpes 134
high blood pressure 96, 224, 225,
229, 233, 236, 243
High Fliers Sweets for Anxious Fliers 90
Holy Sleep Pillow 129
Homage to Hildegarde Hangover Cure 88
Homemade Tiger Balm 89
honey 19, 21, 127
Honey & Marigold Graze Remedy 78
Honey, Lemon & Ginger for Colds 63
hormonal imbalance 114, 224, 228, 229, 230, 243
horse chestnut 31, 95, 224
Horse Chestnut & Broom Varicose Vein Lotion 95
horseradish 157, 174, 226
Horseradish Sauce 157
Horseradish Vodka 174
Horses' Anti-fungal Hoof Paint 138
Horses' Wart Remedy 138
horsetail 230
Hot Cayenne Tincture for Chilli Hot Chocolate & More 156
Hot Oil 155
Hot Stuff Circulation Stimulant 95
hot sweats/flushes 113, 229, 238, 241
House Protection Charm 218
'HRT' cream 113
huang qi *see* milk vetch
huang qin 238
huckleberry *see* bilberry
hyperactivity 233, 234, 236
Hyssop Cough Syrup 64

I

ice cream 159
ice pops/lollies 87, 130, 131
Immune Booster for Horses 138
immune system 55, 163, 174, 226, 227, 230, 232, 235, 241
impotence 115
incontinence 107, 230
Incontinence Tea 107
indigestion 101, 102, 133, 235, 243
   see also digestion; gut; stomach

infertility *see* fertility
infused oils 20
infusions 15
double infusion 18, 20
inks 214
insect bites 89, 92
insect repellents 38, 44, 50-1, 91, 92, 196, 220, 221
insomnia *see* sleep
Intensive Eye Serum 183
Intensive Skin Repair Balm 80
intertrigo 181
Intestinal Parasite Suppositories 103
Intestinal Parasite Treatment 104
intestinal parasites 104, 225, 226, 227, 233, 236
   see also worms
Invigorating Body Butter 187
iron tonic 56
Irritable Bowel Tincture Mix 102
irritable bowel syndrome (IBS) 53, 102, 225, 235
itching 82, 111, 118
Ivy-leaved Toadflax Sandwiches 148

J

jelly 158
Jewellweed Salve for Skin Infections 86
Joint-Aligning Salve 117
joints 57, 72, 116, 117, 170, 230, 231, 240
Juniper, Rosemary & Lavender Glass Cleaner 30

K

Kidney-strengthening Tea 63
kidneys 63, 166, 224, 225, 226, 236, 237, 239, 240, 241, 242
stones 163, 226, 233
kit 16-17, 23
Krishna 39, 235

L

labelling 22
Labour Endurance Mix 112
   see also childbirth

Ladies' Lovelies 108
lady's mantle 224
Lamb's Quarters Herbal Salt 146
lavender 30, 41, 42, 50, 73, 129, 134, 180, 181, 189, 200, 210, 212, 217, 233
Lavender & Rose Handcream 189
Lavender & Rosemary Moth Repellent 50
Lavender & Sage Deodorant Powder 212
Lavender Handwash 200
Lavender-infused Oil 73
Lavender Laundry Soap 41
Lavender Toner 180
Lavender Water 134
laxatives 238, 240, 242
Leafu Protein Supplement 57
leathers, fruit 56
legs 95–6, 191
lemon balm 134, 164, 234
Lemon Balm Vinegar 164
Lemon Balm Water 134
Lemon Barley Water 166
Lemon Boot Polish 215
Lemon-fresh Cleaner 27
Lemon Furniture Polish 32
'Lemon Sherbet' Rehydration Remedy 93
Lemon Zinger Floor Cleaner 30
lemonade 53, 167
Lichen, Coltsfoot & Thyme Cough Sweets 100
liniments 20
Linseed Rehydration Tea 52
lip balm 192
lipsticks 193
Liquid Castile Soap 199
liquorice 65, 161, 232
liver 61, 102, 105, 165, 175, 225, 226, 227, 228, 229, 231, 232, 233, 234, 235, 236, 237, 238, 239, 240, 242
pets 138
lobelia 234
lovage 167
Love Spell Bath Salts 186
Love Spray 37
lucid dreaming 226

lungs 76, 79, 80, 161, 225, 226, 232, 236, 238, 239, 240, 241, 242, 243
Luxurious Body Butter 188
Luxury Laundry Liquid 43
Luxury Moisturizing Handwash 200
Luxury Shaving Cream for Women 212
Luxury Soap 198
lymphatic system 164, 231, 232, 236, 243

M

Mabon Welcome Cup 173
make-up 193
malaria 93, 226, 227
Mandarin Handwash 200
Mange Treatment for Animals 135
Many Berry Cordial 55
Many Berry Fruit Leather 56
marigold 12, 29, 78, 81, 228
marjoram 12, 26, 235
marsh mallow 76, 101, 117, 161, 225
Marsh mallow Cough Syrup 76
Marsh mallow Sweetmeats 161
Marsh mallow Water for Acid Indigestion 101
mascara 193
massage oils 72–4
mastitis 139
meadowsweet 127, 231
Meadowsweet Anti-diarrhoea Honey 127
measurements 18, 23, 103
Medicated Tooth Powder for Gum Disease 210
Medicinal Lavender Skin Tonic 181
Medicinal Mouthwash & Gargle 210
Medicinal Port Brandy 174
memory loss 134, 231
menopause 108, 113, 114, 224, 229, 230, 234, 238, 241, 243
Men's Reproductive Tonic 115
menstruation 108, 109, 110, 114, 165, 224, 229, 234, 240
Mess of Greens 154
Metal Polish 34
migraine 88, 229

milk thistle 105, 239
Milk Thistle Liver Protector 105
milk vetch 59, 227
Milk Vetch, Ginseng & Nettle Stress-support Tonic 59
Mineral-rich Seaweed Bath 62
Mint Chocolate Face Pack 178
Moisturizing Working Hand Scrub 201
Moisturizing Shaving Cream for Men 213
morning sickness 111, 234, 243
Morning Sickness Sweets 111
Mosi Spray 91
mosquitoes 91, 93
Moth-destroying Spray 51
moth repellents 50–1
Mother of the Heart Tincture 75
motherwort 234
mouse deterrent 219
mouth freshener 159
mouth infections 227
Mouth Ulcer Cure 85
mouth ulcers 79, 85, 237
pets 137
moxibustion 226
mucus 80, 124, 125, 127, 224, 226, 238, 239, 242, 243
Mucus-busting Tea 127
mucous membranes 224, 236, 239
mugwort 165, 217, 226
mullein 77, 86, 242
Mullein Flower Oil for Earache 86
Mullein Pile Ointment 77
Multi-mineral Powder 58
multiple sclerosis 231, 232
muscles 72, 74, 89, 117, 155, 165, 230, 234, 240, 243

N

Nail & Cuticle Booster 190
nails 122, 190, 197, 230
Natural Mascara 193
Nature Smoothie 152
nausea 100, 101, 235, 243
navelwort 241
nephritis 239
nervous system 226, 228, 231, 238,

239, 242
nettle 59, 108, 151, 170, 205, 220, 241
Nettle & Sage Shampoo for Greying Hair 205
Nettle & Wild Garlic Lentil Soup 151
Nettle Beer 170
Nettle Syrup 108
night sweats 113
Nit-deterring Conditioner 206
Nit Treatment for Kids 132
No Stress Raw Chocolates 109
nose 79, 238, 239
Nourishing & Cleansing Face Mask 179
Nourishing Nail Oil 190
Nutty Plantain Snack 143

O

Oak Bud Remedy for Strength 71
Oak Leaf Wine 177
oats 130, 148, 149, 195, 227
oatstraw 227
Odour-busting Natural Drain Cleaner 32
Old-fashioned Furniture Polish 33
olive oil 20, 80, 198
onion 76
Opening & Clearing Snuff 124
Orange, Lime & Grapefruit Conditioner 206
oregano 12, 165, 235
Oregano Vinegar 164
Oregon grape 228
oven cleaner 28
oxymels 19

P

pain relief 88, 89, 228, 233, 236, 237, 241, 243
pakoras 145
pancakes 144
papaya 104
parasites *see* intestinal parasites; worms
passion flower 236

Passion Spray 37
Pear & Nutmeg Brandy 172
pennywort 146, 148, 241
Pennywort Sandwiches 148
Pennywort Sattvic Tempura 146
peppermint 133, 235
Peppermint Water 133
Period Pain Chocolates 109
Period Pain Tea 110
period pains 109, 110, 114, 224, 229, 243
Pessaries for Thrush 111
pesto 152
Pets' Bedding Fabric Conditioner 49
Pets' Bedding Laundry Liquid 44
Pets' Liver Tonic 138
Pets' Mouth Wash 137
Pharaoh's Flapjacks 142
picking herbs 11, 13
Pickled Ginger 160
piles 77, 232, 241, 242
pine 29, 99, 143
Pine Cookies 143
pityriasis versicolor 86
Plant-based Wax for Raw Wood 34
Plant Power Car Wax 221
plant sprays 220, 221
plantain 142, 143, 236
Plantain Seedy Flapjacks 142
Plum Mead 173
PMT Chocolates 108
poison ivy 86
pokeroot 236
polycystic ovarian syndrome 243
Polyp Snuff 124
port 174
post-natal depression 230
pot marigold *see* marigold
potpourri 39
Poultice for Broken Bones & Strains 84
poultices 19
pre-menstrual syndrome/tension (PMS/PMT) 107, 108, 228, 243
pregnancy 71, 74, 108, 111, 234, 237, 241, 243
Pregnancy Tea 71

Primrose & Violet Lemonade 167
Probiotic Breakfast 140
Probiotic Lemonade 53
Prosperity Spray 38
Prosperous House Charm 219
prostate 115, 239, 241
Protection Smudge Stick 217
Protection Spray 38
protein supplement 57
psoriasis 43, 119, 201, 228, 232
Psoriasis Cream 119
Psoriasis Lotion 119
Psoriasis Ointment 119
Psoriasis Skin Scrub 201
pumpkin seeds 115
Pungent Pakoras 145
Pungent Pest Control Spray for Plants 220
Pure Liquorice 161
Pure Olive Oil Castile Soap 198-9
Purification Bath Salts 186
purple coneflower *see* echinacea
purslane 160

Q

Queen Anne's Lace Jelly 158
Quick Chamomile Eye Poultice for Sore Eyes 79
Quick Onion Cough Syrup 76
Quick Wake Up 71

R

Radharani's Favourite Ice Cream 159
radiotherapy 122, 227, 230, 235
Radiotherapy Healing Salve 122
Rainbow Potpourri 39
Ramsons Vinegar 163
Rash Ointment 130
raspberry 237
red clover 147, 157, 203, 241
Red Clover Mild Shampoo 203
Red Clover Syrup 157
reflux 102
rehydration 52, 93, 127
Relaxation Bath Salts 186
Relaxing Massage Oil 72
Relaxing Mix for Labour 112

reproductive organs 230, 236
respiratory problems 98, 224, 229, 234, 235, 241
Revive Facial Mist 188
rheumatism 62, 67, 238, 240
ribwort 85, 236
Ribwort Poultice for Infected Wounds 85
ringworm 86
Roasted Reed Rhizomes 155
rob 159
room sprays 36–8
rose 48, 115, 134, 147, 165, 167, 180, 181, 182, 185, 189, 207, 215, 237
Rose & Cashew Cream 147
Rose & Chamomile Water 134
Rose Petal Beads 215
Rose Vinegar 165
Rosehip C Syrup 54
Rosehip, Hawthorn & Pine Throat Lozenges 99
rosehips 54, 55, 99, 237
rosemary 29, 30, 31, 50, 134, 149, 167, 204, 208, 237
Rosemary & Horse Chestnut Scouring Powder 31
Rosemary & Lovage Lemonade 167
Rosemary & Pine Toilet Cleaner 29
Rosemary & Poppy Seed Oatcakes 149
Rosemary Vinegar 208
Rosemary Water 134
Rosy Bath Bomb 185
Rosy Lotion 182
rowanberry 55, 143, 158
Rowanberry Bitters to Stimulate Digestion 143

S

Saffron & Rose Tea 167
sage 84, 97, 205, 210, 212, 216, 217, 238
Sage & Daisy Poultice for Bruises & Swellings 84
Sage & Lavender Deodorant 210
Sage & Lavender Smudge Stick 217
Sage & Thyme Gargle 97

Sage Smudge Stick 216
St John's wort 83, 232
St John's Wort Oil 83
salad 153
salts 146, 147
Salve for Dry Joints 117
Salve for Eczema 126
Sandalwood Deodorant 211
sandwiches 147, 148
Sarcoids Cream for Horses 139
Savoury Pancakes 144
scars 237
sciatica 229
scouring powders 31
Scratch Pet Flea Remedy for Cats & Dogs 136
scrubs 185, 201, 202
seaweed 62, 185
sepsis 227
Sesame & Lavender Baby Oil 129
shampoo 196, 202–5
shaving cream 212, 213
sherry tonic 67
shingles 232, 234
Siberian ginseng 230
silica 230
Simple Rose Face Cream 181
Simple Turnip Cough Syrup 80
Sinus-clearing Inhalation 98
Sinus-clearing Soup 150
sinuses 96, 98, 150, 225, 226, 238
Sinusitis & Infected Teeth Mix 96
skin 49, 57, 66, 69, 72, 74, 80–4, 86, 118, 119, 120, 122, 126, 130, 134, 164, 165, 201, 202, 225, 226, 228, 229, 230, 231, 232, 233, 234, 237, 238, 239, 240, 241, 243
    personal care 178–89
Skin-calm Fabric Softener 49
Skin-calm Tea 118
skullcap 238
sleep 37, 70, 114, 128, 129, 177, 218, 227, 233, 234, 236, 242
Sleepy Tea 70
Sloe Vodka 173
sloes 19, 53, 173
smudge sticks 216–17
snuff 124

soaps 21, 40–1, 194–9, 221
Soapwort Shampoo for Blondes 202
Soapwort Shampoo for Dark Hair 202
Soapwort Shampoo for Redheads 203
Soapwort Wool Wash 46
Solomon's Bad Back Salve 117
Solomon's seal 116, 117, 236
Solomon's Seal & Agrimony Tension Remedy 116
Soothing & Refreshing Foot Bath 191
Soothing Face Mask 179
Soothing Oat Bath 130
Soothing Sloe C Syrup 53
Soothing Snuff 124
Sore Throat Gargle 128
    see also throat
soups 150–1
Space-clearer's Washing Powder 45
Space-clearing Spray 36
spasm 103, 229, 230, 233, 234, 240, 243
Special Baby Wipes 131
Spiced Hawthorn and Rowan Berry Jelly 158
Spicy Elder & Bilberry Rob 159
Spicy Furniture Polish 33
Spicy Laminate & Wooden Floor Cleaner 35
Spicy Laundry Liquid 43
Spray for Strained or Sore Throats 79
stain remover 47
sterilizing 17
stevia 12
Stimulating Massage Oil 72
Stinging Nettle String 220
    see also nettle
stomach 87, 88, 92, 100, 101, 102, 134, 161, 225, 226, 228, 231, 232, 235, 237, 239
    pets 136
    see also digestion
Stone Floor Soap 30
Stop Itch Cream 82
storing herbs 13, 16
strains 84

stress 59, 70, 73, 109, 177, 226, 228, 230, 232, 234, 235, 242
Stress-busting Massage Balm 73
Stretch Mark Prevention Oil for Pregnant Women 74
stroke 231
Sugar & Spice Body & Shampoo Bar 196
sugar cravings 231
sunburn 134
sunscreen 132
Super Anti-cellulite Oil 192
Super-green Juice 56
Super-strong Citrus Washing Powder 45
suppositories 101, 103
sweating 87, 113, 226, 238, 243
Sweet & Soft Fabric Conditioner with Rose 49
Sweet Flower Sandwiches 147
Sweet Kiss 193
Sweet Pickled Purslane Stems 160
Sweet Rose Hair Oil 207
Sweet Sleep Pillow for Children 128
Sweet Sleep Syrup 128
sweets 21–2
swellings 84
Swiss Gentian Aperitif Wine 175
syrups 21
Syrupy Menopause Mix 113

T

Tea for Dizziness 114
Tea Tree & Lemon Deodorant Powder 211
teas 15
teasel 116
teeth 79, 96, 127, 209, 210
 pets 137
teething 127, 225
Teething Rub 127
tempura 146
tension 116, 224, 242, 243
Teri's Tooth Powder 209
throat 53, 64, 76, 79, 87, 97, 99, 128, 210, 238, 239, 241
thrush 110, 111
thyme 12, 29, 31, 65, 97, 100, 240

Thyme & Liquorice Cough Syrup 65
Thyme & Marigold Disinfectant 29
Thyme Disinfectant Scouring Powder 31
thyroid 232
tiger balm 89
tinctures 18–19
 recreational 172–5
Tobacco and Tea Tree Plant Spray 221
toilet cleaner 29
toners 180
tonsils 164, 237
tooth powder 209, 210
toothpaste 209
toothwort 156
Travel Sickness Sweets 90
Travellers' Anti-bug Laundry Soap 40
travellers' first aid kit 90–3
Tree Power Antiseptic Aftershave 213
Tropical Body Buff 184
Tropical Hair Milk 207
true Solomon's seal *see* Solomon's seal
Truly Tasty Cough Mixture 99
turmeric 64, 229
Turmeric Honey Antibiotic 64
turnip 80
typhus 227

U

udders 139
Ulcer-healing Honey 79
ulcers 224, 225, 230, 231, 232
 see also mouth ulcers
Up All Night & Still Dancing Snuff 124
Uplifting Snuff 124
urinary system 225, 232
 see also bladder
urticaria 134

V

vaginal thrush 110, 111
valerian 115, 135, 242
Valerian & Catnip Cat Toy 135
Vapour Rub 98

varicose veins 95, 96, 191
Vein-building Complex 96
veruccas 121
vervain 242
Very Berry Mead 173
Vinegar Calcium Tonic 57
vinegars 19, 163–5, 208
violet 123, 167, 243
Violet Salve for Tumours 123
vitamin C 53, 54, 55, 67, 108, 158, 173, 182, 237, 238
Vitamin E Rich Healing Salve for Animals & People 139
Vitamin Ice Lollies 130
vodka 18, 78, 173, 174

W

wall pennywort 241
walnut 59, 177, 216, 233
Walnut Flower Remedy for Adapting to Change 59
Walnut Leaf Wine 177
Walnut Protection Remedy 216
Warm the Bones Smoothie 62
Wart & Verucca Zapper 121
warts 121, 138, 229, 240
washing liquid 48
washing powder 45–6
washing-up liquid 28
Waterfall Smoothie 107
Waterproofing Mix for Canvas 215
Weight Loss Spice 60
Weight Loss Tea 60
white cedar 240
white willow 237
whitener 47
whooping cough 229
Wild Cherry Cough Calming Syrup 125
Wild Garlic Bread 152
Wild Garlic Pesto 152
Wild Greens 156
Wild Herb Savoury Cream 147
wild indigo 227
wild lettuce 233
Wild Toothwort Sauce 156
wild yam 113, 230
willow 88, 204, 237

255

Willow Shampoo for Oily Hair 204
wind 53, 102, 163, 243
Wind-reducing Syrup 102
window cleaner 30
wines 175, 176–7
Winter Festivities Potpourri 39
Winter Warmer Tea 62
Wintertime Facial Toner 180
womb 71, 134, 224, 226, 227, 234, 237, 243
Women's Balancing Tea 114
wood betony 239
Woodash Detergent-free Washing Liquid 48
wool wash 46
Worm Suppositories 103
worms 103, 240
    see also intestinal parasites
wormwood 226
wounds 78, 85, 224, 228, 232, 233, 234, 236, 238, 240, 241, 242

X

Xmas Survival Tummy Tonic 87

Y

yarrow 96, 170, 179, 224
Yarrow Beer 170
Yarrow Soothing Skin Wash 179
Yellow Dock Crackers 149
yellow jasmine 103

Z

Zesty Stain-remover 47
Zesty Washing-up Liquid 28
zinc 115

ACKNOWLEDGEMENTS

I would like to thank the many people who have made this book possible.

A huge thank you to all at Leaping Hare, particularly the lovely Monica Perdoni, who spotted me during my two-minute *Countryfile* appearance and had the idea for *The Domestic Alchemist*, and Jayne Ansell, who is a tirelessly patient editor. Also thanks to the art director, Wayne Blades, and designer, Andrew Milne, for making a beautiful book.

Thanks to my parents, Sheila and David Waller, who got me into herbal medicine in the first place by their example, and for all their help and support over the years.

Thanks to my beloved Dauji for his loving support and clever suggestions, my son Alex and my friends who tried a lot of weird and wonderful recipes – some that made it, some that didn't! – and listened to a lot of gnashing of teeth as I wrestled with the computer over this project.

Thanks to all the fabulous herbalists, plant spirit medicine practitioners and plant lovers who generously gave their recipes – you have made this book the interesting and varied mixture of recipes that it is. Thanks also to those whose recipes were too long for this volume – I'm hoping to feature yours in volume two!

Thanks to Louise for letting me loose with my cups and spoons in the Herbarium shop and helping me get to grips with US/European measuring eccentricities.

Thanks to my friends in the plant world, the herbs themselves, for calling to me again and again and waving to me wherever I go.

And last but not least, thank you Radharani, for being the One who is behind everything.